PSYCHIATRY – THEORY, APPLICATIONS AND TREATMENTS

EMOTIONALITY, INTIMACY AND TRAUMA OF INTELLECTUALLY DISABLED CLIENTS WITH SELF-HARM, AGGRESSION, DISTURBING BEHAVIOURS AND/OR EMOTIONAL FLUCTUATION (SADE)

HUMANISTIC INTERPRETATION AND INTERVENTION

PSYCHIATRY – THEORY, APPLICATIONS AND TREATMENTS

Additional books and e-books in this series can be found on Nova's website under the Series tab.

PSYCHIATRY – THEORY, APPLICATIONS AND TREATMENTS

EMOTIONALITY, INTIMACY AND TRAUMA OF INTELLECTUALLY DISABLED CLIENTS WITH SELF-HARM, AGGRESSION, DISTURBING BEHAVIOURS AND/OR EMOTIONAL FLUCTUATION (SADE)

HUMANISTIC INTERPRETATION AND INTERVENTION

KAM-SHING YIP

nova
Medicine & Health
New York

Library of Congress Cataloging-in-Publication Data

ISBN: 978-1-53615-280-7
Library of Congress Control Number: 2019936817

Published by Nova Science Publishers, Inc. † New York

Contents

PREFACE

Intellectual disability has long been a concern for both practitioners and academics in recent decades. Within the introduction and advocacy of concepts of normalisation and social role volarisation, humanistic concern for people with intellectual disability became the dominant trend in providing interventions and services for people with intellectual disability. Later, various concepts of inclusion are introduced. Nevertheless, many practitioners and academics criticised that all these concepts are idealistic and, in many ways, inapplicable to actual social inclusion for people with intellectual disabilities. The situation is particularly serious in working with those intellectually disabled clients with various forms of self-harm, aggression, disturbing behaviours and emotional fluctuation (SADE: S = Self harm, A = Aggression, D = Disturbing behaviours, E = Emotional fluctuation). Facing all that, most scholars and practitioners tend to use social control and behavioural management in dealing with these clients. All these are moralised and justified in terms of *behavioural management of challenging behaviours.* The term *behavioural management* is misused to cover out inhumane social control. In actual situations, many practitioners intend to engage in five major control measures. First, a verbal threat is given by practitioners to clients to deter or cease their self-harm, aggression, disturbing behaviours and emotional fluctuation. Second, if clients' SADE continue, social exclusion in forms of time out and social labelling is given to clients. They are labelled as troublemakers and disturbing the logistics and normal flow of activities and pattern in the service. Third, punishment is given in forms of deprivation of rights. For example, if clients do not cease their SADE, practitioners may deprive them of their right to go out for tea, to have home leave or being visited by relatives. In some occasions, physical restraints, such as restricted chair, straitjacket or loading or weights, are given to clients with SADE, particularly those with aggression. Finally, if all these fail to work, clients with SADE are forced to take psychiatric medication. Threat, social exclusion and labelling, punishment and deprivation of right and physical restraints as well as psychiatric medication are commonly used in controlling intellectual disabled clients with SADE. The concept of normalisation and social inclusion seems not to be applicable in actual clinical practice with clients with complicated SADE natures. In many ways, people with intellectual disabilities are regarded as objects of problematic behaviours and emotions that need to be assessed, controlled and managed. Institutionalised abuse in terms of threat, punishment, physical restraints, inappropriate medication and deprivation of rights are common in professional practitioners in service delivery for clients with intellectual disability. All these maltreatments are well-moralised and justified in terms of challenging behaviours and behavioural control. Related practitioners do not have patience, genuine concern and empathy to understand clients' needs, emotion, meaning, function and purpose behind their self-harm, aggression, disturbing behaviours and emotional fluctuation (SADE).

A thorough understanding on those intellectually disabled clients review that their SADE is closely related to their unfulfilled needs, developmental traumas, tortures, abuse, neglect and abandonment and problems in expressing their views and emotions, as well as severe attachment needs. There is a serious shortage of appropriate references and conceptual underpinnings in addressing the need of humanistic, normalised and inclusive practice for intellectually disabled clients with SADE. Based on the writers' years of substantial experiences of clinical practice and supervision in working with intellectually disabled clients with SADE, this book is the first book in the global academic and professional field to provide a normalised, humanistic and inclusive interpretation and intervention for persons with intellectual disability with self-harm, aggression, disturbing behaviours and emotional fluctuation.

The whole book consists of several chapters. Chapter 1 is a shifting of paradigm from inhumane control on challenging behaviours to a deep, normalised, empathic understanding of SADE (Self-harm, Aggression, Disturbing behaviours, and Emotional fluctuation). Various forms of social control challenge behaviours, such as threat and social isolation.

In fact, the term 'SADE' literally means every intellectually disabled client with self-harm, aggression, disturbing behaviours and emotional fluctuation actually has a 'sad' story behind them. SADE are only conscious or unconscious manifestations of all these unpleasant memories, unfulfilled psychosocial needs and emotional complexes within this sad story in a client's life development.

Chapter 2 is a deep and comprehensive articulation of the SADE model. In fact, a deep articulation of clients' SADE showed that there are five levels of articulation. The first level is that 'behaviours in context', all self-harm, aggression and disturbing behaviours should be understood in terms of details, content, process and related physical and psychosocial context. The second level is 'person in context'. That means, in what ways the client feels and thinks during SADE. Related professionals should have an empathic stand in understanding clients' emotions, cognition, meaning, needs, function and purpose behind SADE. Level 3 is 'person in life narration'. In this level, related professionals have to construct a detailed life narration of clients, including happy and unhappy events in infancy, childhood, adolescence, youth, adulthood and aging. Once this life narration is constructed, related professionals can construct in what way the SADE is influenced by related life experiences. Level 4 is 'persons in different life spans'. That means, in what ways the past happy or unhappy experiences and memories are being triggered and recalled by related persons, issues and objects within SADE. Level 5 is 'meaning of flowing in different life spans'. That means, the trigger and recall of past happy and unhappy experiences and memories has special meaning and function for the clients with intellectual disability in the process of SADE.

Also, clinical experiences showed that the occurrence of SADE is closely related to communication and emotionality, intimacy and traumas of clients with intellectual disability.

Chapter 3 is a comprehensive review of emotionality and communication of clients with intellectual disability. Because of limited intelligence, many of them have problems in communication and emotionality. As people with normal intelligence, they also have unresolved emotional complexes in facing suffering, conflicts and hardships in life. However, their limited intelligence and communication ability limits their expression of emotionality, in particular in unresolved emotional complexes. Thus, they may use SADE as ways to release their unbearable emotional complexes, strong negative or intense positive emotions. In clinical practice, behind self-harm may be unresolved anger and hatred feeling towards self. Underlying aggression may be intense anger towards others. Similarly, disturbing behaviours may represent a need to relate to other because of intense loneliness. Emotional fluctuation simply implies unexpressed emotional complexes leading to drastic mood changes.

Chapter 4 is comprehensive articulation of intimacy and attachment needs of clients with intellectual disability. Because of limited intelligence and exposure to opportunities in life, many of them need to depend on caregivers. Comparatively speaking, their intimacy and attachment needs are more intense than people with normal intelligence. However, because of overwhelming caregiving, many family caregivers fail to fulfill clients' intimacy and attachment needs. Some even abandon them or put them in boarding school, residential care or day care centre even though they are very young. Many of them stay in all these services for their whole lives. Home leave or union with their family members becomes a luxury in their daily lives. Most of them earnestly need to have intimate contact with others. They easily regard caregivers in service units as substituted attachment figures. Their attachment hunger easily expresses in forms of disturbing behaviours. However, many workers may regard these as challenging behaviours and try to ignore them. As a consequence, attachment hunger prevails and transforms into self-harm and aggression. This situation is particularly serious for those intellectually disabled clients facing sequential loss of attachment figures. Various intervention strategies to fulfill clients' intimacy and attachment needs in different service units are also thoroughly discussed.

Chapter 5 is a comprehensive discussion of trauma and oppression of clients with intellectual disability. Because of various reasons, many clients with intellectual disability with physical or psychological abuse by caregivers in families and service units. Because of their limited intelligence and communication ability, they are unable to express or communicate all these traumatic experiences and memories. Instead, all these are being dissociated and repressed. However, they can be easily triggered by incoming stimulus. When all these traumatic experiences and memories are recalled and rebounced, with clients' limited intelligence and communication deficit, they can only express all these in forms of severe SADE, in particular, self-harm and aggression.

Chapter 1

A Shifting of Paradigm from Inhumane Control on Challenging Behaviour to Deep, Normalised, Empathic Understanding of SADE (Self-Harm, Aggression, Disturbing Behaviour and Emotional Fluctuation)

Introduction: A Review of Normalisation

Mental retardation and intellectual disability has long been a concern for both practitioners and academics in recent decades. Within the introduction and advocacy of concepts of normalisation and social role volarisation, humanistic concern for people with intellectual disability became the dominant trend in providing interventions and services for people with intellectual disability. Bank-Mikkelsen introduced the concept of normalisation in a piece of Danish legislation called the 1959 Mental Retardation Act.

He described normalisation as a means to ensure people with intellectual disabilities the right to the same community-based existence as their peers without disabilities, including clothing, housing, education, work, and leisure.

In 1971, he became the director of the Department of Care and Rehabilitation of the Handicapped, Danish National Board of Social Welfare, and he was instrumental to the 1980 formation of Denmark's Central Committee on the Handicapped. In the Mental Retardation Act (1959), he described normalisation as 'letting the mentally retarded obtain an existence as close as possible to that of everyone else' (Bank-Mikkelson, 1959).

'A sense of existence' implies a sense of being and continuous existence. 'As close as possible as everyone' means everyone as his/her own sense of existence. 'The sense of existence' of everyone should be unique, continuous and on a reality basis with relationships with others.

Nirje (1969) defined the normalisation principle as 'making available to the mentally retarded patterns and conditions of everyday life which are as close as possible to the norms and patterns of the mainstream of society' (p. 181).

The normalisation principle reflects several perspectives (Nirje, 1993):

1. People with disabilities ought to have lives that are similar to the lives of people without disabilities. Thus, the principle is rooted in the concept of equality.
2. People with disabilities ought to have the opportunity to create and pursue good lives that are related to their own personal situations. Thus, the principle is rooted in the concept of quality of life.
3. People with disabilities ought to be valued and have the same rights as people without disabilities. Thus, the principle is grounded in the concept of human rights.

He identifies eight features of the principle:

1. A normal rhythm to the day during which you do similar things at similar times to those being done by others in society but also with the flexibility that other people take for granted in their day-to-day lives;
2. A normal routine to life, that is to say, living in one place, attending school or going to work in another and participating in leisure activities in yet more places; this also means that people with disabilities have to learn to cope with unexpected, unstructured situations without panicking;
3. A normal rhythm to the year, going on holidays, in some cases abroad, and celebrating birthdays and anniversaries;
4. Experiencing the normal developmental experiences of the life cycle, such as a stimulating environment in the care of a few significant adults during childhood, opportunities for learning about one's own personal abilities and potentialities, for obtaining understanding of oneself and for building self-confidence in youth, the experience of being accepted, treated and respected as an adult, including the opportunity to start a life of one's own, as independently as possible and the opportunity to spend one's old age in familiar settings as close as possible to those with which they have been acquainted as adults;
5. Having one's choices, wishes and desires taken into consideration and respected, something which is facilitated by opportunities to express oneself within small groups;
6. Living in a bisexual world where there are both male and female staff and acceptance that wanting to get married and to live together are normal;
7. As normal economic standards as possible, for example, drawing the same benefits as anyone else even where these may have to be topped up and being paid an economic wage for work done; and
8. Standards of facilities similar to those others are accustomed to, for example, accommodation no larger than that which other people would occupy as a long-term residence in locations similar to those of other forms of accommodation (Nirje, 1969: 185-7).

In 1972, Wolfensberger defined normalisation as follows:

'The use of means which are culturally normative to offer a person life conditions at least as good as the average citizens and to, as much as possible, enhance or support personal behaviors, appearances, experiences, status, and reputation….To the greatest degree possible ….At any given time….For each individual according to his or her developmental needs'. (Wolfensberger, 1972: 23)

Wolfensberger (1972) further elaborated the definition as follows:

'The use of means….' The ways in which people are helped are just as important as the help itself. For instance, there are many ways to teach skills. One skill that we might want to teach a child or adult is pouring. One way to teach children is in a sandbox with pails and shovels; but adults should be taught the same skill through cooking lessons or potting plants.

'….which are culturally normative….' The principle of normalization applies to all societies, but what is 'normative' or 'typical' in one society may not be 'normal' or 'typical' in another.

'….to offer a person life conditions that at least as good as the average citizen's….' This refers to income, housing, health care, social resources, and opportunities – the material basis of everyday life. Anything we would not accept, we would reject at the outset for people with special needs.

'….as possible….' These words are important. There are limits to what is possible, and normalization does not demand the impossible. It does, however, demand that we test the bounds of the possible.

'….enhance or support personal behaviors, appearances, experiences, status, and reputation….' We are working toward enabling people with developmental special needs to learn to appear, to behave, and to act in ways which our society would consider typical or desirable. For instance, only a few people in our society live in large communal groups – learning, working, sleeping, and eating in the same building.

> Most people dress and groom themselves with a sense of style. Adults and many children learn to use public transportation and to shop in the community. Yet many people who have special needs have never had these opportunities.
>
> *'....to the greatest degree possible....at any given time....according to his or her developmental needs....'* Each person is constantly growing and changing. In order to help in the future progress or development of a person, we need to understand what that person can do now. If the help is below or too far beyond the actual place where the person is, miseducation and injury may result. But for everyone there is a place to start and a lifelong capacity to continue to learn. (Wolfenberger, 1972: 53)

All these showed that normalisation is a widely adapted ideology in rehabilitation services in which people with intellectual disability should be regarded as normal as other people. They should enjoy the same right, opportunity, daily pattern, respect and dignity as all normal people.

Social Role Valorisation (SRV) is the name given to a concept for transacting human relationships and human service. Wolfensberger's (1985) definition of SRV is:

> 'The application of what science can tell us about the enablement, establishment, enhancement, maintenance, and/or defense of valued social roles for people'.

The major goal of SRV is to create or support socially valued roles for people in their society, because if a person holds valued social roles, that person is highly likely to receive from society those good things in life that are available to that society, and that can be conveyed by it, or at least the opportunities for obtaining these.

In other words, all sorts of good things that other people are able to convey are almost automatically apt to be accorded to a person who holds societally valued roles, at least within the resources and norms of his/her society (Osburn, 1998:7).

NORMALISATION: MYTH AND REALITY

Challenges or Burden of Normalisation in Clinical Practice

It is clear all these well-defined ideologies of normalisation became an international trend in affirming that every person with intellectual disability should be fully respected and enjoy the same rights as other normal people in society. Despite normalisation being well-developed concepts with refined discussions of service delivery, facilities, policy implementation and advocacy, related literature rarely discusses clinical practice with clients who are intellectually disabled, in particular, those with behavioural, emotional and mental problems. In clinical practice, the implementation of normalisation has many burdens and challenges. Firstly, most clients with intellectual disability have communication problems; their needs and emotions cannot be fully communicated to others. Related caregivers, especially those frontline workers, easily ignore their unexpressed needs and emotions. It is common that related professionals and frontline workers impose their own biases and assumption on clients.

Secondly, clients with intellectual disability, particularly those who are severely and profoundly disabled, are highly dependent on others. Caregivers, including family members and personal-care workers, may not have enough patience, empathy and genuineness to understand, to interact and to communicate with clients with intellectual disabilities. Related caregivers, including related professionals in various service units, are inclined to maintain a regular flow of daily activities and schedule for every client with intellectual disability within the same service units. In many cases, to ensure a rigid division of labor, accountability and efficiency of the regular flow of daily activities and schedule in the service unit may gradually become more and more rigid, that is, similar to features of a total institution as mentioned by Goffman.

Thirdly, despite many professionals and frontline workers having heard and even being trained regarding normalisation, quality of life, inclusion and person-centred approach, they rarely learn about humanistic orientation in interpretation and intervention of intellectual disabled clients with self-harm, aggression, disturbing behaviours and emotional fluctuation. In fact, apart from behavioural therapy and modification, scholars and practitioners in other perspectives, such as psychodynamic, existential, phenomenological, social and cognitive approaches, do not show much interest in clinical practice on clients with intellectual disabilities, especially those with SADE. The deficit in theoretical underpinning easily makes related professionals feel helpless, confused in facing severe SADE and inclined to control with medication.

Fourthly, in recent years, quality control and assurance, evidence-based practice as well as cost-effectiveness analysis pushed related professionals to accountability-based practice rather than a client-centred understanding, connection and interaction-based intervention. Intellectually disabled clients with SADE are easily labelled as troublemakers, disturbing the regular flow of daily activities and schedule. Self-harm and aggression need to be stopped immediately by directive, coercive and emergent measures.

Partial Normalisation and Dichotomisation of Normalisation and Abnormalisation

Because of above-mentioned challenges and burdens, clinical practice in intellectually disabled clients with SADE are easily abnormalised as troublemakers that need to be controlled, punished or restrained or as sick persons who need medical treatment. The concepts of normalisation has become dichotomised. For those intellectually disabled without SADE, or those complied and social ones, they are advocated to be normal people. They are encouraged to have various kinds of life opportunities, exposures and training. Some may have special skills such as creative art, sports and music. Some may be selected as representatives in advocacy groups for people with intellectual disabled. Some have distinctive performances in work, education and social contribution. In society, equal opportunities, accessibility to community facilities and anti-discrimination ordinance are fully advocated. Normalisation is fully actualised to 'good', 'social', 'smart' and 'distinctive' people with intellectual disabilities. However, to those intellectually disabled clients with SADE, normalisation is being neglected. Instead, abnormalisaton is applied. As SADE is abnormal, clients need abnormal treatment, such as restraint, punishment, medication and hospitalisation.

Normalisation is not only dichotomised to intellectually disabled clients with SADE, it is also partially applied. Most academics, practitioners and policy makers only care about normalisation in a collective sense rather than applying to individual client with intellectual disability, especially those with SADE. Normalisation is only applied to those intellectually disabled in a 'normal' condition. That is, normal in social interaction, normal in complying to regular flow of activities and schedule in service units, normal in following caregivers' instructions and normal in the ability in expression one's own ideas, views and emotions.

CHALLENGING BEHAVIOURS: MORALISATION OF INHUMANE INSTITUTIONAL CONTROL OF SADE

Goffman's Characteristics of Total Institution

Goffman (1957) points out the following characteristics of a total institution (asylum), such mental hospitals and prisons. They are listed as follows:

Rigid Daily Activities, Schedule and Pattern

1. All aspects of life are conducted in the same place and under the same authority.
2. Each phase of the member's activities well-conducted out in the immediate company of a large batch of others all whom are treated alike and required to do the same thing together.

3. All phases of the day activities are tightly scheduled, with one activity at a prearranged time into the next. The whole circle of activities are being imposed from above through a system of explicit formal rulings and a body of officials.
4. Finally, the contents of various enforced activities are brought together as parts of a single overall rational plan purportedly design to fulfill the officials aims of the institution.
5. The handling of many human needs by bureaucratic organisation of whole block of people; whether or not this is a necessary effective means of social organisation is a key fact of the total institution.
6. Block of people move in time to use a relatively small number of supervisory staff.

Split of Inmates and Staff

1. There is a basic split of a large number of inmates and a small number of supervisory staff.
2. Each group tends to conceive of members of the other in term of narrow hostile stereotypes.
3. Staff often seeing inmates as bitter, secretive and untrustworthy, while inmates often see staff as condescending, high-handed and mean.
4. Staff often feel superior and righteousness; inmates tend to in the same way feel inferior weak, blameworthy and guilty.
5. Social mobility between the two strata is grossly restricted, social distance is typically great and often formally prescribed and even talk across the boundaries may be conducted in a special tone of voice.

Mortification of Privilege and Punishment System (Summarised)

1. There is a mortification in which shame was induced to inmates through a privilege and punishment system.

2. There is a set of rigid rules and regulations imposed and designed by supervisory staff to inmates.
3. Those who follow these rules and regulations will be rewarded by the privilege system in terms of materialistic rewards or non-materialistic rewards in terms having rights to community visits, meetings with visitors or home leave.
4. Those who violate these rules and regulation will be punished by the punishment system in terms of restrain, isolation, deprivation of rights or even physical punishment or abuse.
5. The mortification will be moralised and justified for the smooth running of the institution, good of clients and actualisation of ideologies and values of the institution.

Definitions and Types of Challenging Behaviours

Definitions of Challenging Behaviours

Challenging behaviours, also known as behaviours which challenge, are defined as '*culturally abnormal behaviour(s) of such intensity, frequency or duration that the physical safety of the person or others is placed in serious jeopardy, or behaviour which is likely to seriously limit or deny access to the use of ordinary community facilities. Ordinarily we would expect the person to have shown the pattern of behaviour that presents such a challenge to services for a considerable period of time. Severely challenging behaviour is not a transient phenomenon*' (Emerson, 1995: 3).

Challenging behaviour used to be called 'problem behaviour', 'difficult behaviour' or 'socially unacceptable behaviour'. It means that behaviours are a challenge to professionals, teachers, carers and parents. A person with challenging behaviour is not a 'problem' to be fixed and is not doing something 'wrong'. But behaviour is a sign that something isn't working. It shows that there is some unfulfilled need or a problem with communication. Behaviour is challenging if it causes harm or if it stops people fulfilling some aspect of their lives (Scope about Disability, 2010).

Types of Challenging Behaviours

Challenging behaviour can be:

- Self-injurious: Head-banging, scratching, pulling, eye-poking, picking, grinding teeth, eating things that aren't food.
- Aggressive: Biting and scratching, hitting, pinching, grabbing, hair pulling, throwing objects, verbal abuse, screaming, spitting.
- Stereotyped: Repetitive movements, rocking, repetitive speech and repetitive manipulation of objects.
- Non-person directed: Damage to property, hyperactivity, stealing, inappropriate sexualised behaviour, destruction of clothing, incontinence, lack of awareness of danger, withdrawal. (Scope about Disability, 2010)

Abusive Control of Challenging Behaviour in Clients with Intellectual Disabilities

From Challenging Behaviours to Behaviours of Concern

Chan et al. (2012) affirmed that the term *challenging behaviours* is misused and abused by related professionals in intervention and service to client with intellectual disability. Royal College of Psychiatry et al. (2007) says in facing challenging behaviours, related professionals should understand underlying psychosocial and physical causes and prevent them from recurring. Restriction and punishment should be avoided in the process of service delivery and intervention. The term 'challenging' in fact refers to a threat to related professionals that demand they response immediately to the safety of clients and others. It is administratively defined rather than a profound understanding the underlying contextual and personal factors (Chan, et al. 2012). It is easily used by related professionals in stereotyping and labelling of clients with intellectual disability. Although it is innovatively suggested by Emerson (1995), it is increasing recognised as depowering to clients with intellectual disabilities and frequently misused and abused by related professionals and frontline workers in imposing institutional abuse (Chan et al., 2012). They suggest another term 'behaviour of concern' to replace the term 'challenging behaviours'. They also suggest that there are various causes underlying 'behaviour of concern' including mental-health conditions, relationship problems, deficits in social support network and breakdown of communication as well as context problems.

Five Measures in Misuse and Abusive Control on Clients with Challenging Behaviours

Challenging behaviours are usually SADE. Intellectually disabled clients with challenging behaviours are commonly abusively controlled by related professionals and caregivers. The writer had carried out an action research for nine years in helping related professionals learn how to properly and humanely support more than three hundred intellectually disabled clients with SADE. Without a humanistic, empathic and normalised orientation, related professionals and frontline workers are inclined to engage in the following five measures to control/manage challenging behaviours in terms of SADE.

The First Measure Is Threat

It can be a verbal threat, physical threat or eye threat. Threat is different from prompting. Underlying threats are caregivers' and related professionals' senses of unresolved anger, helplessness and frustration. Threat is a means to release all this anger, helplessness and frustration. In prompting, caregivers and professionals are emotionally and psychologically confident and peaceful with attention on helping to enhance clients' sense of reality and awareness of their harmful behaviours. In addition, threat usually implies order, control on clients to cease SADE immediately or else punishment will be imposed. Verbal threat means that the client was verbally warned by frontline workers. Physical threat implies physical posture, which implies a possible insulting or humiliating punishment that may be imposed on clients if they fail to stop challenging behaviours immediately. Eye threat refers to threatening looks or stares with a full angry and punitive manifestation. Verbal, physical and/or eye threats means related professionals and caregivers are assuming challenging behaviours are abnormal, unacceptable and unbearable. Interestingly, in real practice, many challenging behaviours, in particular disturbing behaviours such as continuing to make noises, trying to pull and getting close to certain workers and strong attachment behaviours, do not involve any safety problems. Nevertheless, physical, verbal and eye threats are commonly imposed by related workers to clients.

The Second Measures Are Stereotype and Labelling

Very often, clients with frequent challenging behaviours in terms of SADE are being labelled by related workers and caregivers as troublemakers. They are, in fact, challenging the authority of workers, challenging the regular flow and scheduled activities in the service units and making them spend extra time, effort and attention. That means, challenging behaviours force related workers and caregivers to come out from their normal or comfort zones in the daily duties. So, clients with SADE should be labelled as troublemakers. Their challenging behaviours should be stopped to reduce their extra time, effort and attention needed. The more the service units are institutionalised, the stronger is the labelling and stereotyping should be imposed on the troublemaking clients. Certainly, individual clients with SADE create a strong disturbance to highly rigid activities and schedules in which blocks of clients collectively move from one daily activity to another one. For example, an individual client who fails to eat any meal as his/her favourite worker is being transferred to another table to serve another group of clients. S/he manifests strong attachment behaviours to this worker by dumping food on his/her table and tries to eat food from another table. Within the framework of challenging behaviours, the client's attachment need is ignored. Instead s/he is labelled as a troublemaker having aggression and disturbing the scheduled arrangement of mealtime and making related workers spend extra effort and time to clear up the dumped food and restricting him/her to come to another table.

The Third Measure Is Restriction, Restraint and Isolation

Within the stereotyping and labelling process, related professionals and caregivers are moralised and justified to impose restriction, restraint and isolation to clients with challenging behaviours in terms of SADE. The above-mentioned client with strong attachment needs is labelled in terms of attention seeking. The more s/he struggles to attach to his/her favourite worker at mealtime, the more related professionals are moralised to isolate him/her from this worker. An intellectual disabled and autistic client with frequent self-harm because of unexpressive pain of being rejected or abandoned by his/her parents will be restricted on a seat in a restricted jacket to stop all these self-harm behaviours. The deep-seated pain of being abandoned by parents is totally ignored in the process of management. Very often, most workers in the service unit are not conscious or aware that a client's self-harm is related to early abandonment or self-hatred feeling in the development process. Underlying restrictions, restraint and isolation are intense abnormalisations of clients with challenging behaviours. Together with this is a strong urge of related professionals to demonstrate their dominance and exercise their power. In using restraint, restriction and isolation, most professionals are moralised with an institutionalised attitude as mentioned by Goffman (1957) that clients (inmates) are controlling, manipulating and trying to break the rules and regulations; thus, punishment should be imposed on them. On the mind of highly institutionalised workers, communication and understanding of clients with challenging behaviours is useless and a waste of time. For these clients are abnormal, unreasonable, controlling, rebellious and manipulating. Only by means of this moralisation can related workers cover up their own senses of dominance, control, superiority and helplessness in working with clients with challenging behaviours.

The Fourth Measure Is Deprivation of Rights of the clients with challenging behaviours. As mentioned by Goffman (1957), most institutionalised service units have a clear system of privilege and punishment. Those clients following rigid daily schedule and activities are classified as good and complied ones. They are rewarded by having the right to go outside, have home leave, join the community and have recreational activities. Those clients with challenging behaviours in terms of SADE are deprived of all these rights. They are punished by not being allowed to go outside, to have home visits, or join related communities and recreational activities. Deprivation of these normal rights are, in fact, psychological abuse and emotional abuse being imposed on vulnerable clients with challenging behaviours. However, within the moral justification for the quality of life of all clients in the institutionalised service units, this type of psychological abuse and emotional neglect is covered up in terms of efficient management of challenging behaviours.

The Final Measure Is Inappropriate Medication and Hospitalisation

In clinical practice, many clients with challenging behaviours are influenced by prolonged neglect and abandonment from caregivers, poor communication and the inability to express their deep-seated negative emotions. The more they are deprived of these normal rights, the more they feel frustrated and the more severe will be the challenging behaviours. As the four measures – threat, stereotyping, restriction and deprivation of rights – cannot reduce challenging behaviours but rather intensifies them in terms of frequency, intensity and duration, related professionals tend to label clients as having mental problems that need the treatment of psychiatrists. In some cases, hospitalisation is implemented to remove the real troublemakers from the service unit to a mental hospital, in particular those with aggressive behaviours. Clinically speaking, there is no psychiatric medication to reduce self-harm, to cease aggression or to treat disturbing behaviours. Thus, in actual practice, aggression is similar to psychotic confusion that anti-psychotic medication, such as Risperdal, is commonly imposed. Self-harm is similar to depression in which an antidepressant such as Prozac. Inappropriate or overuse of psychiatric medication is common and regarded as final measures for clients with challenging behaviours. Upon the writer's nearly ten years in supervising professionals in working with intellectually disabled clients, despite taking a high dosage of psychiatric medication, challenging behaviours in terms of SADE still prevail. However, instead of challenging the treatment effects of psychiatric medication, related professionals tend to continue inappropriate psychiatric medication. Many professionals and caregivers are inclined to adhere to the following misbelief in medication:

1. It is better to use medication rather than rely on humanistic understanding and psychosocial intervention in facing challenging behaviours in terms of SADE.
2. It is better to continue those medications previously taken rather than changing the type and dosage. Related clients not only have a long history of medication but also taking more and more types and dosage of psychiatric medication.
3. Medical professionals, in particular psychiatrists, are final and the highest authority in managing or treatment of clients challenging behaviours, despite having the least time in encountering and least understanding of related clients.

In facing intellectually disabled clients with severe aggression, apart from psychiatric medication, involuntary hospitalisation is imposed. Unfortunately, the process of involuntary hospitalisation in forms of coercive restraint, the use of a straitjacket is a traumatic experience for the client. It further aggregates the client's fear and flight defence. The more the client is involuntarily hospitalised, the more the client is traumatised, the more s/he is sensitive to others' physical touch and holding and the more the client is irritated and defensive. As a result, the client becomes more aggressive.

Moralisation of Maltreatments of Challenging Behaviours

Interestingly, the five measures in imposing abusive control on clients with challenging behaviours in terms of SADE are institutionalised physical restraint, psychological abuse and emotional neglect imposed by related professionals and caregivers. However, all this abusive control is moralised and justified. There are several mechanisms in moralisation and justification. The first mechanism is interpreting abusive control as behavioural management. Instead of having a good training on behaviour therapy in terms of refined observation, proper articulation of intensity, frequency and intensity, details, process and context of individual challenging behaviour, related professionals and caregivers simply justify and moralise their five measures of abusive control as behavioural management. They wrongly regard threat as prompting, letting clients beware of they are going but in fact, they are threatening them. They try to justify isolation as time-out in behavioural therapy. They interpret their physical restraint as for the safety of other clients and staff. They moralise their labelling and stereotyping as assurance of normal flow of regular schedule and activities. Finally, the privilege and reward system are according to the rigid and institutionalised house rules as well-structured behaviour modification strategies.

The Second Mechanism Is Medicalisation

Related professionals and caregivers, as mentioned above, simply put the final accountability of clients' challenging behaviours on psychiatrists and medical practitioners in which they believe medication and hospitalisation is the final and most professional way to deal with clients' challenging behaviours in terms of SADE.

The Third Mechanism Is Accountability

Related professionals and caregivers affirm that threat, stereotyping, physical restraints, medications, hospitalisation and deprivation of clients' rights are proper and efficient measures to cease challenging behaviour for the sake of protecting other clients' and staff's safety. They regard all challenging behaviours in terms of SADE as unexplainable, not understandable, without any psychosocial causes, but they simply are crisis, risks and emergencies. Thus, threat, stereotyping, physical restraints, medications and deprivation of rights are proper measures in crisis intervention and emergency management. They may elaborate this in forms of a working manual to manage clients' challenging behaviours in the service units.

Shifting the Paradigm from Institutionalised Abusive Control to Humanistic Understanding and Intervention

From Abnormalisation to Deep and Profound Normalisation

Clinical practice in intellectually disabled clients with challenging behaviours in terms of SADE are easily abnormalised as troublemakers that need to be controlled, punished or restrained or as sick persons with medical treatment. The concepts of normalisation become dichotomised. For those who are intellectually disabled without SADE, or those complied and social ones, they are advocated to be normal people. For those with SADE, abnormalisaton is applied. They should be abnormally threatened, stereotyped, restrained, isolated, and medicalised and hospitalised. Thus, for a humanistic understanding and intervention for clients with SADE, deep normalisation and profound normalisation is needed. *Deep normalisation* despite clients with self-harm, aggression, disturbing behaviours and emotional fluctuation, they are still normal people. In clients with underlying abnormal challenging behaviour, or SADE, there are unexpressed normal positive or negative emotions, problems in normal communication and interaction and unfulfilled normal needs of being loved and cared for, as well as unexpressed and untreated of traumatic experiences and memories of being neglected, abandoned and abused. *Profound normalisation* implies profound tolerance of client's frequent, intensive and durable self-harm, aggression, disturbing behaviours and emotional fluctuation and avoids imposing threats, deprivation of rights, physical restraints, medication and hospitalisation on clients. Related professionals and caregivers should believe that challenging behaviours are an unhealthy coping of deprivation of normal love, concern and care, normal way of communication and expression of deep-seated positive or negative emotions, as well as manifestation and adjustment of traumatic experiences and memories. Only by facilitating clients to fulfill all these normal needs, clients' SADE will be gradually reduced and diminished. For a full recovery from challenging behaviours, normal intervention and environment is needed to establish clients' normal, meaningful and healthy sense of existence, self-esteem, personal competence, life satisfaction and life pattern.

From Challenging Behaviour to Behaviour of Concern and Positive Behaviour Support

Despite challenging behaviour being innovatively suggested by Emerson (1995), it is increasing recognised as depowering to clients and frequently misused by workers imposing institutional abusive control. Chan et al. (2012) suggest 'behavior of concern' to replace the term 'challenging behaviors'. They also suggest that there are various causes underlying 'behavior of concern' including mental-health conditions, relationship problems, deficits in social support network and breakdown of communication as well as context problems (Chan et al., 2012). Carr et al. (2002) advocated for the term 'positive behavior support' (PBS). They define PBS as follows:

> PBS is an applied science that uses educational methods to expand an individual's behavior repertoire and systems change methods to redesign an individual's living environment to first enhance the individual's quality of life and, second, to minimize his or her problem behavior.
>
> Positive behavior includes all those skills that increase the likelihood of success and personal satisfaction in normative academic, work, social, recreational, community, and family settings.

> Support encompasses all those educational methods that can be used to teach, strengthen, and expand positive behavior and al l those systems change methods that can be used to increase opportunities for the display of positive behavior. (Carr et al., 2002:4)

In other words, PBS's first focus is on clients' skills and abilities to live a better life. Problem behaviours is only a second priority and instead of imposing abusive social control, clients are facilitated to achieve his/her needs and goals in a socially acceptable manner (Carr et al., 2002). PBS emerged from three major sources of ideologies:

a. Applied behaviour analysis,
b. The normalisation/inclusion movement, and
c. Person-centred values.

It also has several critical features:

- Comprehensive lifestyle change and quality of life,
- Life-span perspective,
- Ecological validity,
- Stakeholder perspective,
- Social validity,
- System change and multicomponent intervention,
- Emphasis on prevention,
- Flexibility with respect to scientific practice, and
- Multiple theoretical perspective.

That means, PBS tries not to label or stereotype the client. Instead, it focuses on a person in environment orientation. The interpretation of challenging behaviour should not be a victim-blaming orientation. Instead, it should be a multidimensional orientation with behaviour in context, person in context and person in life span.

From Threat to Communication and Emotional Connection

Within the abusive control of challenging behaviours, threat is used. Underlying threats are caregivers' and related professionals' senses of unresolved anger, helplessness and frustration. Threat is a means to release all this anger, helplessness and frustration. While related professionals release their own negative emotions. they tend to neglect clients' emotions in challenging behaviours in terms of SADE. Ross and Oliver (2002) affirmed that intellectually disabled adults' challenging behaviours may be related to their depressive or negative moods. In fact, most clients with intellectual disabilities may have problems with communication and expression of negative emotions. In clinical practice, behind self-harm may be unresolved anger and hatred feeling towards self. Underlying aggression may be intense anger towards others. Similarly, disturbing behaviours may represent a need to relate to other because of intense loneliness. Emotional fluctuation simply implies unexpressed emotional complexes leading to drastic mood changes. Thus, instead of imposing a physical threat, related professionals and caregivers should first ensure clients with challenging behaviours in terms of SADE and be well-communicated. They should try their best to facilitate clients' unresolved negative emotions behind their challenging behaviours. In doing so, workers should be highly empathic and sensitive to clients' cognition and emotion behind their challenging behaviour, as well in their past experiences.

From Isolation to Attachment and Intimacy

Very often, for clients with intellectual disabilities, underlying their challenging behaviours in terms of SADE is a strong attachment need. Instead of stereotyping clients as manipulative, attention seeking, destructive and disturbing and imposing isolation and restraint, it is important to cater to clients' unfulfilled attachment needs in various ways continuously. Clinically speaking, self-harm can be an expression of anger towards oneself as being abandoned by significant others. Aggression can be a displacement of anger of being abandoned by others. Disturbing behaviours can be a manifestation of strong attachment needs. Within an empathic stance, related workers and professionals should interpret clients' challenging behaviours in relation to their intimate and attachment needs. Janseen, Schuengel and Stolk (2002) have done a comprehensive review on research on stress and coping as well as on the security of the attachment relationships of people with intellectual disabilities. There is evidence that people with intellectual disabilities are more vulnerable to stress and use less-effective coping strategies. Furthermore, the body of studies on attachment indicates that people with intellectual disabilities are at risk for developing insecure, especially disorganised, attachment (Janseen, Schuengel and Stolk, 2002: 445).

From Physical Restraint to Trauma Orientation

Physical restraints are commonly used by related professional and caregivers in facing clients' challenging behaviours. In some cases, involuntary hospitalisation is enforced, particularly in facing clients' aggression. All these are moralised and justified by crisis intervention and psychiatric emergencies. Within an abusive control orientation and institutionalised service contexts, crisis, emergency and safety are only concern and orientation. Within an empathic stance, related workers should shift from a crisis orientation to a trauma orientation in perceiving and interpreting clients' challenging behaviours in terms of SADE. Crisis orientation and trauma orientation are different in the following ways:

Crisis Orientation

1. Sudden and intensive negative events;
2. Out of individual's coping and management;
3. Crisis can be tided over;
4. Individual can resume ability and status quo before crisis;
5. Each crisis is singly existing; and
6. Boiling down individual emotion so as to adapt the crisis rationally.

Trauma Orientation

1. Can both be predictable or unpredictable;
2. Can be single events or accumulated episodes and repeated events;
3. Trauma can be tided over but the traumatic memories and harm can be lifelong;
4. Individual's status quo is changed by the trauma;
5. Traumatic memories and traumas can be easily triggered, provoked and irritated by clues in environment; and
6. Acute stress disorder or dissociation and dissociated traumatic memories can be rebounced in the form of post-traumatic symptoms.

Within a trauma orientation, clients' challenging behaviours may be a conscious or unconscious response in terms of dissociation, triggering, rebounce and/or dissociation of traumatic memories and experiences in life developmental process. In some cases, institutional service and abusive control of challenging behaviours are harmful interventions. These interventions are service-induced traumas to clients, which can further intensify and exaggerate SADE.

The Humanistic SADE Interpretation and Intervention

Within an empathic stance, and basic result of action research on five different rehabilitation service agencies and clinical practice on more than three hundred intellectually disabled clients with SADE, the writer has constructed a humanistic SADE model. In fact, the term 'SADE' literally means every intellectually disabled client with self-harm, aggression, disturbing behaviours and emotional fluctuation actually has a 'sad' story behind them. SADE are only conscious or unconscious manifestations of all these unpleasant memories, unfulfilled psychosocial needs and emotional complexes within this sad story in a client's life development.

The writer will describe this model in detail in the coming chapter. This model consists of several components:

The first component is ideology. It based on deep and profound normalisation in which clients with SADE should still be considered as normal people with unfulfilled needs, hidden and unresolved emotions, as well as happy and unhappy past experiences. *The second component is detailed observation and analysis of SADE.* It can be incidental and just happen once for all (*incidental SADE*). It can be highly patterned occurring in a stable and regular format (*pattern SADE*). It can be highly patterned and occur in a severe and intense manifestation (*Severe SADE, SSADE*). It can be obsessive and severe and patterned (*severe and obsessive SADE, SOSADE*). *The third component is psychosocial causes of SADE.* It can be a matter of miscommunication between clients and others (usually in incidental SADE). It can be a matter of improper release of unresolved emotions (usually in pattern SADE). It can be a matter of expression of attachment hunger and intimacy need (usually in severe SADE, SSADE). It can be a matter of unconscious rebounce or repression of traumatic memories and experiences (usually in severe and obsessive SADE, SOSADE). *The fourth component is levels of interpretation and understanding.* Level 1 is behaviours in context, in what way SADE occurs within different physical and social contexts. Level 2 is person in context, in what way the client with SADE feels, thinks and responds to external stimuli. Level 3 is person in life narration, in what way SADE is related to the client's own life experiences. The fourth component in fact embraces a complication of a systemic view of persons in environment as well as a client life narration.

CONCLUSION

As a conclusion, this chapter is an overview of related ideologies in rehabilitation of clients with intellectual disabilities, followed by a comprehensive critic of challenging behaviours in terms of SADE. Challenging behaviours is an innovative term recently proposed by

Emerson (1995) but increasingly misused by related professional for abusive and institutionalised control of clients with intellectual disabilities. It easily nurtures various kinds of abusive control, such as threats, stereotyping, isolation and restraints and deprivation of rights, as well as inappropriate medication and hospitalisation. Furthermore, all these abusive controls are further moralised and justified by crisis intervention, emergencies, accountability and behavioural management. For humane professionals with a full belief of normalisation, there should be a paradigm shift from abusive control to humanistic interpretation and intervention of challenging behaviours in terms of SADE. Related professionals should shift from abnormalisation and partial normalisation to deep and profound normalisation, from threat to humanistic understanding and emotional connection, from isolation to attachment and intimacy, from physical restraints to trauma orientation. Finally a humanistic SADE interpretation and intervention model is constructed by the writers' clinical experiences and action research. In the next chapter, a comprehensive articulation of the SADE model is described.

Chapter 2

A Deep and Comprehensive Articulation of the SADE Model: From Behaviours in Context, Person in Context to Person in Life Narration

Introduction: An Innocent Institutionalised Mental Patient with Intellectual Disability

Intellectually disabled clients with challenging behaviours in terms of SADE are commonly abusively controlled by related professionals. For those with aggressive or self-harm behaviours, they are involuntarily hospitalised and are forced to take psychiatric medication, even though they do not have any psychiatric problems. In some cases, some are institutionalised in mental hospitals for many years. Below is a case illustration of this maltreatment. Related parties' consensus to use their stories are sought. For the sake of confidentiality, personal information and identities are properly disguised.

R was adult client with an intellectual disability. He was born in a middle-class family in which his father was a teacher and his mother was a clerk in a shipping company. R had an elder brother and a young sister. In R's mother's pregnancy, related tests showed that he might suffer from an intellectual disability. His father insisted R's mother undergo an abortion but she refused. As a committed Christian, she wanted to keep R. Thus, the giving birth of R became a conflicting issue between his parents. After R was born, despite that he was intellectually disabled, he appeared to be a lovely baby.

Two years later, R's sister was born. His mother quit her job as a full-time housewife to take care of R. Later, R's father was promoted as the headmaster in a primary school. While R's mother tried her best to take care of R, his father felt shameful to have a son with moderate grade of intellectual disability. Emotionally, he detached from R. He did not accept R as his son. At home, he avoided talking and playing with R. Even though R's mother tried her best to encourage a father–son relationship, he was inert, passive and withdrawn in interacting with R. Occasionally, if R did anything wrong at home, his father might become furious and impose physical punishment on R. At that moment, R's mother would come up and defend him. Because of that, R's parents had intensive quarrels about the caregiving of R. It made R very frustrated.

Despite that he was intellectually disabled, he fully acknowledged that he was rejected by his father. Facing all that, R harboured intensive anger towards his father as well as towards himself. However, because of his limited intelligence, indeed, it was really hard for him to express all these complicated feelings. Instead, whenever, his father was present, this unresolved anger was triggered. To release his anger, he hit and bumped his head hard and frequently. Whenever his mother saw this, her heart was broken. She came forward and embraced R not to do so. However, her husband insisted that R was silly, retarded and hopeless and should be institutionalised in an asylum. When R heard that, he was so sad. He cried bitterly and bumped his head even harder. His mother was so sad and helpless in facing R's self-harm. Also, her husband pushed her very hard to put R into a boarding school for clients with intellectual disabilities. Finally, R was put into a boarding school.

He stayed there for eight years. During this period of time, R's self-harm behaviours intensified. He bumped his head in the boarding school whenever he felt puzzled, confused and angry. Instead of understanding R's feeling behind his self-harm behaviour, R was labelled as emotionally unstable. The social worker in the boarding school referred R for psychiatric treatment. Instead of understanding R's deep-seated self-directed anger in facing the rejection of this father, the psychiatrist simply diagnosed R as having psychosis and required him to take antipsychotic medication. From that time onward, R was required to take antipsychotic medication. However, it did not help much for him to lessen his self-harm behaviour. Spontaneous bullying and isolation from his teachers in the boarding school made R not only committed in self-harm behaviours but also aggressive behaviours towards others. Whenever others rejected or bullied him, he might suddenly rush to the bully and bite him/her. After that, he would go to the bathroom and bump his head on the bathroom wall.

All these self-harm and aggressive attacks threatened both teachers and social workers in the boarding school. The frequency and intensity of self-harm and biting others increased gradually. Very often, R would harm himself severely causing bleeding on his head. He also bit others seriously when he felt angry and confused. Related caregivers could do nothing to deter all these self-harm and aggressive behaviours. Caregivers in the boarding school tied R's hands whenever he tried to perform self-harm or aggressive behaviours. Finally, with his mother's consensus, R was admitted to a mental hospital. From that time onwards, R was hospitalised. R was frustrated by that. To ventilate his anger of being abandoned and detained in the mental hospital, at first, R was irritated and committed even more intensive self-harm and aggressive behaviours. Because of that, he was restrained in his bed for two days to deter self-harm and aggressive behaviours. In addition to that, he was injected with a heavy dosage of antipsychotic medication. Soon, all this made R became dull, inert and passive.

From R's case, it was clear that R was totally misunderstood by related parties including his parents, his teachers and medical professionals. They tended to neglect R's intense urge to be attached and accepted by his father.

They did not understand that R could not copy well with his father's rejection. They seemed to assume that R was intellectual disabled; thus, he did not have feelings of sadness and frustration as others did. They interpreted R's self-harm and aggressive behaviours simply as mental and emotional problems induced by intellectual disability. Instead of understanding the symbolic meaning and emotional needs behind all these self-harm and aggressive behaviours, they simply regarded them as mental problems that should only be solved by continual psychiatric medication. Interestingly, even if R's self-harm and aggressive behaviours became worse, even after continual medication, they still insisted that continual medication as well as hospitalisation was the only way to manage and control R's self-harm and aggression.

In this chapter, the writer attempts to have a comprehensive description of the SADE levels of interpretation and intervention.

LEVELS OF SADE: A HUMANISTIC AND MULTIDIMENSIONAL INTERPRETATION AND INTERVENTION

Within a humanistic articulation, there are different levels of interpretation of **s**elf-harm, **a**ggression, **d**isturbing behaviours and **e**motional fluctuation (SADE). The result of this writer's action research showed that there are altogether five levels of interpretation starting from Level 1 behaviour in context to Level 2 person in context to Levels 3, 4 and 5, a focus on clients' life narrations. Different levels imply different orientations forming a comprehensive and multidimensional framework in articulation of clients with SADE. It is a gradual process in which related workers can move from behaviours to context, from behaviour to person, and from person to life narration. It is a three-dimensional conceptual frame guiding individual worker interpretation and intervention. The first dimension is environment and context in which the SADE happens. The second dimension is moving behaviour to the client's own inner world during SADE. The third dimension is multidimensional towards the client, including the client's meaning of life, self-identity, emotion, cognition, morality and behaviours. It also includes a time dimension, past, present and future. A multidimensional orientation enables related workers to widen their institutionalised attitude, to enhance their empathic sensitivity and to embrace a normalised and inclusive perspective towards clients' SADE.

Level 1: Behaviour in Context

The first level of humanistic SADE interpretation and intervention is behaviour in context. It enables workers to begin their interpretation from a refined and comprehensive articulation of behaviour in SADE. It is a multidimensional behavioural analysis. It includes the following elements:

A. Intensity, frequency and duration of related SADE;
B. Related social and physical context and environment;
C. Related persons, issues, things; and
D. The process, content, details of SADE.

Intensity, Frequency and Duration of SADE

For every behaviour in SADE, its intensity, frequency and duration has strong implications in interpretation and intervention. Intensity means how intense SADE is manifested. Frequency implies how frequent SADE is performed. Duration is how long SADE is done. Very often, related workers fail to a refined observation on the client; they simply impose their own impression on the client's SADE. It is not surprising that different workers may have different interpretations on individual client's SADE. While one labels that it is an aggressive behaviour, another one may presume that it is just a disturbing behaviour. A refined observation of intensity, frequency and duration of individual SADE can clarify all these discrepancies. Aggressive behaviours usually occur in high intensity and low frequency. However, aggressive behaviours occur in high frequency, but low intensity are disturbing behaviours in terms of attachment behaviours.

Related Social and Physical Context and Environment

A good understanding of individual SADE must include related social and physical context and environment. For example, a yelling loudly in an open and wide space is a proper and healthy release of negative emotions. However, a sudden loud yelling in a closed space becomes a highly irritative and disturbing behaviour. Even worse, a loud yelling at the ear of a specific person certainly is aggressive and harmful. Related social environment includes what sort of people are around, what the emotional atmosphere is like and what sort of psychosocial stimuli are being related to SADE. For example, a self-harm behaviour occurring when the client is being bullied or humiliated by workers or other clients is vastly different from self-harm repeatedly occurring in forms of mild self-biting within a boring or anxious mental condition. It is important that related professionals can have a refined recall of related social and physical environment in every occurrence of SADE. If the individual SADE happens in similar social and physical environments, that means external stimuli may be a crucial cause of the SADE. Nevertheless, an individual SADE happening across different social and physical environments may imply insidious and internal causes. Interestingly, an individual SADE happening differently in various social and physical environment implies that the SADE changes to different psychosocial and physical stimuli. All these are important to an accurate and valid understanding and intervention of clients' SADE.

Related Persons, Issues, Things

Related persons, issues and things happening in the process of SADE are crucial in understanding a client's SADE. Individual SADE happening towards a specific person may mean this person triggers the client's negative emotion of unhappy memories. Individual SADE happening towards a group of persons may imply the client is not focussed on the individual person but rather the interaction and dynamics within the group of the person. Issues and things means what exactly happens before, during and after the SADE. It helps workers to have a good empathic understanding of what exactly occurs in the process of SADE. For example, a client's sudden outburst of aggression towards a nearby client is a displacement of anger in current or past experiences. A repeated aggression towards a specific person implies a projection of anger towards this person.

The Process, Content, Details of SADE

All the above enables workers to know about the process, content and details of SADE. Process means what happens, including issues, things, persons, related social and physical environment before, during and after the occurrence of individual SADE. Content implies the substantial act, frequency and duration of individual SADE. Details means any minor and refined details that can be observed in the process of SADE. The more refined the process the content and details of SADE are known to related workers, the more accurate, effective and humanistic the interpretation and intervention will be.

Related Interventions

In according to above-mentioned details of Level 1, a thorough understanding and intervention on SADE should embrace the following:

1. Immediate measures according to related intensity, frequency and duration to avoid exaggeration and unnecessary crisis control;
2. Avoid triggering by related persons, issues and things; and
3. Relate D (process, content, details) to ABC and induce change accordingly.

All these can be illustrated in the following case episodes:

Case episode 1:

> Vincent was a client with an intellectually disability. He was fat, impulsive and had difficulties in verbal and emotional expression. Very often, when he was hurrying to toilet, anyone who hindered his action would be intensely pushed by them. Once, a young, thin female worker hindered his way to the toilet, and he pushed her away. It hurt her. She bumped her head and hurt her forehead deeply. She also twisted her ankle and was sent to the hospital. From that time onwards, Vincent was labelled as impulsively aggressive and violent. He was then on antipsychotic medication.

The case was known to the writer for clinical supervision. After a careful review of his situation, it was identified that his aggressive act was intense, very low frequency and had a short duration. A full understanding of the details, context and process of his aggressive act revealed that it was just an incidental aggression because of difficulties in communication and expression of needs and emotions. Later, after a full training of communication and expression of his needs in going to the toilet, related aggressive acts were diminished. Antipsychotic medication was no longer needed.

> Case episode 2:

> Mary was a client with an intellectual disability. Her parents were well educated and felt shameful to have a daughter with an intellectual disability. When she was only five, she was sent to a boarding school. Her parents rarely allowed her to have home leave. When she was only eighteen, she was sent to a hostel for clients with intellectual disabilities. Mary was, in fact, abandoned by her parents. She harboured strong attachment hunger towards others, in particular a frontline worker who was middle aged, well dressed and looked like her mother. Every time this worker got close to her, she would try to catch her hand, touch her dress or simply cling on her body. Instead of regarding this as an attachment need, this worker interpreted this as attention-seeking, disturbing behaviour and tried to ignore her. The more she was isolated and ignored, the stronger her attachment need became. It also stirred up her abandonment anger. Gradually, her attachment need was intensified

and diffused to other workers as well in forms of mild aggression, such as hitting and pulling others' hair. Finally, she had time out and was isolated by workers. Her mild aggression intensified to strong aggression acts, such as pulling other hairs and tightly clinging to others bodies. She was forced to take antipsychotic medication, but related aggressive behaviours did not have any changes.

The case was known to the writer for clinical supervision. After a careful review of the situation, it was discovered that initially her attachment behaviour manifested in the form of disturbing behaviour with low frequency, low intensity and moderate duration. Gradually, inappropriate and abusive control of challenging behaviour made the disturbing behaviours upgraded to mild aggression with high frequency, moderate intensity and moderation duration. Finally, it became strong aggression with moderate frequency, high intensity and moderate duration. After catering her attachment needs by continuous caring and attended by her substituted attachment figure, her aggression gradually reduced and antipsychotic medication was also no longer needed.

Level 2: Persons in Context

After a good capture of related details in Level 1, behaviour in context, related professionals already embrace a comprehensive understanding of individual SADE. In some situations, a good and comprehensive understanding of Level 1 already implied a good and effective intervention. For a comprehensive understanding and intervention, it is important that related workers have an empathic stance on individual SADE. They should think about how the client thinks, feels and responds in SADE. That is an important shifting from a behaviour orientation and focus on a person. This is also an important change of the client's attitude from challenging behaviours to client performing the behaviour, from threat, control, labelling and punishment to understanding of the client, from abnormalisation to deep normalisation. A good articulation of Level 2 should include the following:

A. Unfulfilled needs,
B. Emotions,
C. Meaning,
D. Function, and
E. Purpose.

Unfulfilled Needs

Unfulfilled needs mean clients' SADE is an expression and manifestation of clients unfulfilled and unexpressed normal needs. It includes physical needs, psychological and social needs. Physical needs may imply preferred food, an urge to eat in time of hunger. It may also include other physical needs such as fatigue, the need to rest, sickness, an expression and release of extra physical energy, sex urge and erotic desires. For example, a male intellectually disabled client with severe autism may be involved in frequent physical stimulation of his penis either by rubbing on others' legs or public self-masturbation, which is certainly an indecent, disturbing or even aggressive behaviour. Underlying this behaviour is an expression of unfulfilled erotic desires, release of intense physical energy or self-stimulation within a highly boring and institutionalised service setting. *Psychological needs* mean a need of recognition, self-actualisation, need of communication and expression, expression need of emotion and recall, affirmation, expression and sharing of cognition and thinking. Some of them are within the client's consciousness. Some may be unconscious. Some may be happy. Some may be unhappy. For example, an intellectually disabled client may harbour a full expectation to be visited by his beloved father once a week and bring him to have tea in his favourite Chinese restaurant. Unfortunately, his/her father fails to do so that week. He then feels sad and angry but displaces his/her anger by hitting and biting his/her roommates. Once the worker promises to bring him to have tea in his favourite Chinese restaurant, his unfulfilled need is fulfilled, and his anger and aggression stops immediately. Social needs mean the need to be loved, cared for, attended to and accepted by others. It also includes having fun, sharing, interacting and having recreation with others. Very often, underlying SADE are various unfulfilled needs. Some are expressive and conscious by the client. Some are unexpressive and unconscious by the client.

Emotion

For every individual SADE, there is underlying emotions, positive or negative. However, because of limited intelligence, they have difficulties in fully expressing, sharing and ventilating these emotions. Instead, they use SADE to express this. For example, an intellectually disabled client eagerly looks for his father's visit in the evening around 5:00 p.m. She is happy but anxious and harbours a strong fear that her father may not able to come. However, her limited communication ability hinders her in expressing all these complicated emotions fully. Because of that, starting from early morning, she frequently asks her workers when her father will come. Even though the worker answers her repeatedly many times that it is around 5:00 p.m., she keeps on asking. Most workers may conclude that she is a highly disturbed and troublemaker. If one worker can facilitate her to ventilate all these complicated emotions by saying that she earnestly hopes for her father visit and is anxious that her father may not come. The worker can also help her to phone her father and make sure he will come. Her disturbing enquiry will reduce and disappear. Similar to people with normal intelligence, clients with intellectual disabilities also harbour unresolved emotional complexes, such as super and inferior complex, approach and avoidance complex, and love and hate complex. SADE is used as a means to express all these unresolved complexes.

Meaning, Purpose and Function

For every SADE, there are its underlying meaning, purpose and function. Underlying self-harm there may be a meaning of 'I am not a worthwhile person to be loved by others, I hate myself'. The purpose of explicit self-harm can be 'no one likes me', or 'do you like me even though I am so worthless'? The function of self-harm can be a complication of self-hate and self-pity as well as getting others' mercy. Similarly, aggression may have a hidden meaning of 'you hate me, I hate you too' or 'you treat me bad, so I attack you'. The function and purpose of aggression can be a self-defence, a projection of anger on others or a displacement of anger towards nearby persons. It is important that related professionals can understand all these hidden and concealed meanings, purposes and functions of SADE.

Related Interventions

Level 2 interpretation of clients' unfulfilled needs, emotions, meanings, purposes and functions of SADE can lead to an effective intervention with the following procedures:

1. Thorough understanding on client's unfulfilled needs, emotions, meanings and functions underlying SADE within related physical and social context;
2. Facilitate clients to have and to construct appropriate and healthy ways to fulfill unfulfilled needs in this context;
3. Ventilate and connect with clients' positive and negative emotions in this context;
4. Healthy way to actualise hidden meanings and life aspirations in this context;
5. Recognise and develop strengths and talents in social functioning in this context; and
6. Appropriate and healthy ways to actualise the hidden purpose in this context.

Level 3: Person in Life Experience and Stories

Importance of Client's Life Narration

Life narration is often neglected by practitioners in clinical practice. Many practitioners simply regard behavioural therapy, cognitive therapy and problem solving as the crux of psychosocial intervention. They think a holistic understanding of clients' life histories is not necessary and time consuming. People with intellectual disabilities, like people with normal intelligence, have their own personalities.

Some are introvert, some are extrovert, some are sociable and some are quiet and silent. They also have their own experiences and memories in life development. Some are happy and enjoyable. Some are unhappy and even full of sufferings and traumas. They also harbour hope and aspirations in life.

All these have continuous influences on one's meaning in life, identity, cognition, thinking, emotions and deeds. Within a normalised, humanistic and holistic orientation, client's SADE is just a manifestation, expression and reflection of all these life experiences and memories as well as socially constructed meaning in life, identity, emotions, cognitions and thinking. It is common for a client with previous experiences of being oppressed and bullied by others in childhood and adolescence to become defensive and aggressive in adulthood. A person with prolonged sufferings and traumas of being abandoned by other harbours intense attachment hunger, abandonment anger and fear, making them become highly sensitive to interpersonal relationships.

A person with a history of being physically abused by others is highly reluctant in physical touch by others. A person who is continuously controlled and demanded by parents in childhood becomes highly anxious and self-demanding in adulthood. S/he is also highly vulnerable to depression and self-introjected guilt.

Life Narration Table

Thus, after the Level 1 (behaviour in context) and Level 2 (person in context) interpretation and intervention, related workers should embrace a life narration perspective on clients with SADE. A life narration should include clients' experience in infancy, childhood, adolescence, youth and adulthood. The table below is a template constructed by the writer in helping professionals to understand the life narration of clients with SADE.

Table. Life Narration of Clients with SADE

Chronological Events in Life	Happy Important Developmental Events in Life (Family, Health, Education, Peer, Employment)	Unhappy Important Developmental Events in Life (Family, Health Education, Peer, Employment)	Related Emotion, Coping, Aspiration, Strengths, and/or Difficulties	Remarks (Analysis and Findings)
Infancy				
Childhood				
Adolescence				
Youth				
Adulthood				
Aging				

Happy and Unhappy Experiences in Life

Within every life stage, for clients with intellectual disabilities, like other people with normal intelligence, they have happy and unhappy experiences.

All these happy and unhappy experiences do not just happen separately, but they intermingle and accumulate with one another. A person loves his wife deeply for many years, and feels extreme loss in facing his wife's death. The deeper and happier his former experiences with his wife, the more painful it becomes in the loss of his wife. Within this line of thinking, unfulfilled needs, emotion, cognition, thinking, meaning, function and purpose underlying SADE should be closely related with happy and unhappy experiences in life.

When related workers have constructed the life narration table for the worker in clinical practice, there are many types of relationships. Below are some of them:

1. A coping and resilience of stress, suffering and trauma in current and past life.
2. A symbolic to recall a happy experience in the past.
3. A triggering and response to trauma and suffering in life.
4. A fixated way to fulfill unfulfilled needs and aspirations.

Dimensions in Life

Apart from these, the life narration table also enables the worker to have an empathic and profound understanding of the client's meaning of life, self-system, personality, emotion, cognition and behaviour patterns. Each dimension of life may consist of the following details:

- Meaning of life (life aspiration, meaning of suffering, life mission, meaning of love, sense of existence, religious thinking)
- Self-system (self-identity, self-image, self-boundary)
- Mind (emotion, cognition, consciousness, morality, reflection)
- Body (health, body image, figure, sexuality, appearance)
- Behavioural pattern (social functioning and role of financial condition)
- Social system (family members, peers, inmates at service units and significant others at various social circles)

Related Interventions

Once the life narration table is constructed, happy and unhappy experiences is known, and various dimensions of life are described. Related workers are able to:

1. Enable significant others to understand that the client's SADE is shaped by their unpleasant or traumatic events in various life histories, in particular abandonment, abuse, neglect and difficulties;
2. Facilitate clients to ease out or ventilate all these deep-seated frustrations in life;
3. Provide good activities, good and supportive significant others and/development to rebuild the client's healthy meaning of life, self-identity, positive emotionality, good social functioning in family, work and education; and
4. If possible, under suitable conditions, provide an intervention to heal clients and their family members.

All these can be demonstrated by the following case illustration. Related parties' consensus to use their stories for academic purpose was sought. For the sake of confidentiality, related identity and personal information is properly disguised.

Case Illustration: The Lonely Water Lover: Allan

Allan was an adult client with intellectual disability and autism. He had been living in a hostel for clients with intellectual disabilities for more than ten years. In residential life, he was lonely, quiet and rarely talked with others. Among workers and professionals in the hostel, he seemed to quite attached to Mary, a kind and caring frontline worker. Occasionally, he liked to engage in some strange behaviours. He would rush to the bathroom and take a quick but intense cold shower. After the cold shower, he did not dry himself. Instead, he returned to his own bed and curled up like a small child for one or two hours. Sometimes, it made Allan feel sick for a few days. Because of that, related workers tried to stop Allan from doing that. However, when Allan intended to do so, anyone who hindered his way would be pushed away. As Allan was physically strong, sometimes it really hurt. Allan was sent to a psychiatrist, and he was labelled as emotionally unstable and aggressive. Antipsychotic medication was given to him for five years. However, Allan's condition did not have any changes. As a clinical consultant for this agency, the writer facilitated related workers to have refined analysis of humanistic interpretation and intervention of SADE. Below are the Levels 1, 2 and 3 interpretations and interventions.

Level 1 Interpretation: Behaviours in Context

A refined observation and recall of Allan's strange behaviours showed that it occurs with a high intensity, moderate frequency and long duration. He took showers with a widely opened water tap. He repeated this behaviour once or twice a month, particularly more in winter. Interestingly, every time before he performed this impulsive behaviour, he was angry and frustrated. There were some conditions that might have led to this impulsive behaviour. Firstly, whenever, he heard that his parents refused to visit him, he felt frustrated and might do this strange behaviour. Secondly, when he asked for the concern of his favourite worker and she refused him, he might feel frustrated and might perform this behaviour. Thirdly, when he was bullied by other inmates and he could not fight back, he felt frustrated. In this level of interpretation, related workers began to figure the whole process, details and content of Allan's strange behaviours. Within this level of intervention, the most important thing was how to connect and help Allan to ventilate his negative emotions of being neglected, rejected and bullied by others. However, in this level of interpretation, related workers were still unable to understand why Allan needed to take a cold show and needed to be wet, making himself sick.

Level 2 Interpretation: Persons in Context

After a thorough discussion with related workers, we began to understand the unfulfilled needs, emotion, cognition, meaning, purpose and function underlying his strange behaviours. It was clear that Allen longed for other love and care, in particular from his parents and his favourite worker. This was why when they rejected or failed to cater to his intimate and emotional needs, he felt frustrated and angry, which led to this strange behaviour. Related emotions of this behaviour are loneliness, anger, fear of being rejected and abandonment. In this level of interpretation, related workers began to understand when Allan took a cold shower, he indeed wanted to cool down himself and release his anger and fear. He refused to dry himself and curled up like a child in bed. This might be a regressive behaviour; he tried to act like an infant so as to earn others' care and love. That means, related interventions should be focused on giving enough care and concern to Allan. If they could provide regular concern and care to Allan, his strange behaviour should be greatly reduced. However, this level of analysis was still unable to understand why the cold shower was chosen to make himself sick.

Level 3 Interpretation: Life Narration

Related workers were encouraged to construct a life narration for Allan. They tried to find happy and unhappy events in Allan's infancy, childhood, adolescence and adulthood. It was found that Allan came from an upper-middle-class family. His mother was a senior teacher in a renowned secondary school. His father was a chief executive in a large international company. They felt shameful in having a son with intellectual disability and autism. All their colleagues' children were smart and bright. Allan also had a younger sister. She was smart, active, brilliant and lovely. Allan's parents tried to focus all their attention on Allan's sister and neglected Allan. They sent Allan to a boarding school when Allan was only six. From that time onward, Allan longed for the concern and care of his parents. They only allowed Allan to come home once a month on Saturday and Sunday. On a long holiday, Allan still needed to stay in the boarding school, and they occasionally visited him. The same thing happened in the hostel. Allan was only allowed home leave once every two months, and his parents only visited him once a month. Every time, Allan's parents connected with related workers, they were quite detached and did not care much about Allan's condition. However, whenever Allan was sick, they were very nervous. They tried to question related workers why they were so careless and let Allan become ill. Sometimes, they even lodged a complaint to this agency about that. It was clear that Allan knew that whenever he was sick, he might be able to get the care and concern of his parents. In this level of interpretation, related workers began to understand the meaning of being sick was a symbolic manifestation of his urge to get the concern of his parents. However, why the cold shower was chosen was still unknown. Related intervention should be focused on how to encourage Allan's parents to have more care and concern for Allan in normal situation rather than merely on his sick time. If Allan's parents fail to do so, Allan's favourite worker should serve as a substitute attachment figure. Further, Allan needed more normal and healthy activities and interaction with other residents. As Allan was quite strong physically, he was encouraged to join a jogging team with a male instructor and ten more clients in this hostel. The male instructor cared for Allan well, Allan felt good, and the frequency and duration of the strange behaviour was greatly reduced.

Level 4: Flowing and Connecting a Client's Life Experiences in Different Periods of Time

Connection and Flowing of Current and Past Experiences

After the Level 3 life narration, related workers began to construct the whole life history as well as how happy and unhappy life experiences relate to individual SADE.

However, to have an accurate and deep understanding, Level 4 interpretation is needed. In fact, consciously and unconsciously, during the occurrence of SADE, the client connects the current situation with past experiences and memories. There can be an overlapping and a comparison of the current and past experiences. For example, a person feels very lonely as he is rejected by his girlfriend. In fact, the rejection is mild and tolerable. However, he compares his whole life of unhappy experiences, such as being abandoned by his mother when he was only five, his father left him when he was ten and then he was then taken care by his uncle and aunt. Unfortunately, he was bullied and oppressed by his nephew. All these negative experiences can be suddenly accumulated together making him feel very sad and angry. This is the reason why he responds very strongly to his girlfriend's mild rejection. He even yells at his girlfriend, cursing at her. For clients with intellectual disabilities, the same thing occurs. That means, when SADE occurs, there are flowing and connection of life experiences and memories in different periods of time.

Different Types of Connection and Flowing

In clinical practice of intellectually disabled clients with SADE, a client's life experience in different periods of time are flowing and connecting in terms of:

A. Negative emotion (inferiority, loneliness, fear and anger);
B. Positive emotion (security, comfort, happiness, competence, togetherness, acceptance) (love, hope and trust);
C. Triggering of trauma or happy memories;

D. Aspiration of life and daily routine; and
E. Fixation of coping and survival mechanism.

Related Interventions

Once clients flowing and connection of life experiences in different periods of time are constructed, related interventions should focus on avoiding triggering of unpleasant experiences, disconnecting current stimulation and past-fixated memories or fulfilling unfulfilled aspirations in life. Related intervention can include the following components:

1. Understanding How this connection and flow is related to clients' SADE;
2. Construct a path as to why clients are being triggered (internal or external or both) in the manifestation of SADE;
3. Explore and develop a client's healthy and positive emotion, event, memory, aspiration and coping in life; and
4. Gradually replace negativity by positivity.

Case Illustration: Water-Lover's Dream

Related workers, after Level 3 interpretation, embraced a good understanding that Allan's strange behaviour should be related to his parents' care and concern attitude during his sick time. Allan's parents were invited to have a chat about Allan's condition. They disclosed the following stories to the workers.

> Allan's parents said that they were also annoyed by his strange behaviours. They did not understand why Allan did so. Once, they brought Allan on a two weeks' trip to a European country in wintertime. They visited several cities, and the whole family enjoyed the holidays very much. However, when they came to a large frozen lake, Allan slept on the ice and refused to get up for an hour, making them very embarrassed and uneasy. Allan caught a severe cold and needed to be hospitalised for a few days in this city. Another time, they visited a fish store, and Allan picked up the ice in the fish store and put it into his clothes.

> They felt puzzled and confused. The writer helped them to recall more refined details and events in Allan's childhood. They finally recalled once Allan got a cold after swimming at a beach for a long time. He had a high fever and needed to be hospitalised. The doctor said that Allan was infected by a serious virus and his health was at risk. They were very anxious and stayed with Allan for a few days until he was away from the critical period.

At that moment, Allan's parents and related workers began to understand why Allan loved to take a cold shower so impulsively. In fact, the memories of being closely taken care of by his parents while having a high fever was so important to him. This was his only memory of being deeply cared for with concern by his parents. As his parents tried to avoid and detach from him and did not accept his intellectual disability, as well as autism, being severely sick seemed to be the only way to earn his parents' care and concern. His parents finally admitted the deepest need of Allan in earning their care and concern. They cried bitterly and admitted their faults of trying to neglect and ignore Allan. From that time onward, they brought Allan home on leave more frequently and regularly. They learnt to embrace Allan and phoned him daily. Coupled with the constant concern and love from related workers, Allan's impulsive cold showers diminished.

Level 5: Making Meaning of a Client's Flowing and Shifting of Life Experience in Different Periods of Time

After Levels 1, 2, 3, and 4 interpretation, most workers nurture a profound and deep understanding of clients' SADE. They become more empathic and caring. They no longer rely on threats, physical restraints, deprivation of rights, stereotyping and inappropriate medication and hospitalisation. Level 5 is a final conclusion in clients with SADE. Related workers should understand clients' meaning flowing and shifting of life experience in different periods of time. Clinically speaking, meaning and connection and flowing can exist in the following forms. The first form is resolving inconsistency in the past and present. In Allan's case, his impulsive cold showers tried to resolve the inconsistency of current parental rejection and neglect and the deep care and concern during his high fever time. The second form is expressing frustration and needs in reality. Within Allan's impulsive act, he also tried to express his deepest anger and frustration in being rejected, bullied and refused by others. The third form is asserting oneself of protection from perceiving incoming threats. For example, whenever a client with an intellectual disability feels frustrated or rejected by others, he will use an umbrella to defend himself by moving the umbrella around in the service unit. Every worker in the service unit labels him as aggressive and violent. After a SADE humanistic multilevel interpretation, related workers finally understand this is only a defensive act. In childhood, the client was abandoned by his parents, and he lived in his uncle's home who did not care about him. Every day he wandered around a nearby park and was constantly bullied by a gang there. To defend himself, he had to fight back with an umbrella. This was the reason why he carried an umbrella everywhere, and whenever he felt frustrated, he would move this umbrella around to defend himself. Apart from these three forms, there are other forms of meaning making, all of them are listed below:

A. Resolving inconsistency in past and present;
B. Expressing frustration and need in reality;
C. Asserting oneself or protection from perceived incoming threat;
D. A continuous or rigid but unhealthy way of coping with frustration;
E. Making meaning of life and manifestation of one's existence;
F. A lifelong defence mechanism; and
G. A means to obtain a substitute attachment.

Related Interventions

After related intervention in Levels 1, 2, 3 and 4, most client's with SADE have recovered. It is necessary to develop healthy and normal life habits, activities and interactions to actualise their self-identities, meaning of life and fulfill their attachment needs. Related intervention strategies are listed as follows:

1. Understand clients' meaning of connection and flowing of different life experiences behind highly patterned SADE; and
2. Explore healthy, normalised means (within similar or different contexts) to resolve inconsistency, expression of frustration, satisfaction of normal needs, self-actualisation, defend of threat and obtain substituted attachments in different social contexts.

CONCLUSION

In conclusion, this chapter is a comprehensive review of different levels of interpretation and interventions of SADE. In fact, a deep articulation of clients' SADE showed that there are five levels of articulation. The first level is 'behaviours in context'. All self-harm, aggression and disturbing behaviours should be understood in terms of details, content, process and related physical and psychosocial contexts. The second level is 'person in context'. That means, in what ways the client feels and thinks during the SADE. Related professionals should have an empathic stand in understanding clients' emotions, cognition, meaning, needs, function and purpose behind SADE. Level 3 is 'person in life narration'. In this level, related professionals have to construct a detailed life narration of clients including happy and unhappy events in infancy, childhood, adolescence, youth, adulthood and aging. Once this life narration is constructed, related professionals can construct in what way the SADE is influenced by related life experiences. Level 4 is 'persons in different life spans'. That means, in what ways, the past happy or unhappy experiences and memories are being triggered, and recalled by related persons, issues, objects within SADE. Level 5 is 'meaning of flowing in different life spans'. That means, the trigger and recall of past happy and unhappy experiences and memories has special meaning and function for the clients with intellectual disabilities in the process of SADE.

In each level, related workers need to be empathic and move closer and closer to clients' inner worlds and life experiences, as well as unfulfilled needs. Related interventions in each level as case illustrations are also given. In the next three chapters, the writer will describe how SADE relates to communication and emotion, intimacy and attachment, as well as traumas and sufferings in clients' lives.

Chapter 3

EMOTIONALITY AND COMMUNICATION OF CLIENTS WITH INTELLECTUAL DISABILITIES: IMPLICATIONS IN INTERPRETATION AND INTERVENTION OF SADE

INTRODUCTION

Emotions, communication and social interaction are crucial in for every human being within every social context. For people with limited intelligence, many of them have problems in communication and emotionality. As people with normal intelligence, they also have unresolved emotional complexes in facing suffering, conflicts and hardships in life. However, their limited intelligence and communication ability limits their expression of emotionality, in particular in unresolved emotional complexes. Thus, they may use SADE as ways to release their unbearable emotional complexes, strong negative or intense positive emotions. In clinical practice, behind self-harm may be unresolved anger and hatred feeling towards self. Underlying aggression may be intense anger towards others. Similarly, disturbing behaviours may represent a need to relate to others because of intense loneliness. Emotional fluctuation simply implies unexpressed emotional complexes leading to drastic mood changes. This chapter is a comprehensive review of emotionality and communication of intellectually disabled clients with SADE. The chapter begins with a description of diagnosis and features of intellectual disability and follows with an overview of communications and emotionality. Then, problems and difficulties of emotionality and communication of people with intellectual disabilities are mentioned. Finally, interpretation and intervention of clients with SADE in terms of emotionality and communication are discussed.

Intellectual Disability: Diagnosis and Feature

Diagnosis Criteria of Intellectual Disability

According to DSM V (APA, 2012), intellectual disability (intellectual developmental disorder) is a disorder with onset during the developmental period that includes both intellectual and adaptive functioning deficits in conceptual, social and practical domains. The following three criteria must be met:

A. Deficits in intellectual functions, such as reasoning, problem solving, planning, abstract, thinking, judgment, academic learning and learning from experience, confirmed by both clinical assessment and individualized, standardized intelligence testing.
B. Deficits in adaptive functioning that result in failure to meet developmental and social cultural standards for personal independence and social responsibility. Without ongoing support, the adaptive deficits limit functioning in one or more activities of daily life, such as communication, social participation and independent living across multiple environments, such as home, school, work and community.
C. Onset of intellectual and adaptive deficits during the developmental period.

Specifiers

The various levels of severity are defined on the basis of adaptive functioning, and not IQ scores because it is adaptive functioning that determines the level of supports required. Moreover, IQ measures are less valid in the low end of the IQ range (APA, 2012: 33).

Severity of ID (Mild Grade)

Conceptual Domain

For preschool children, there may be no obvious conceptual differences. For school-age children and adults, there are difficulties in learning academic skills involving reading, writing, arithmetic, time or money, with support needed in one or more areas to meet aged related expectations. In adults, abstract thinking, executive function (i.e., planning, strategizing, priority setting, and cognitive flexibility) and short-term memory, as well as functional use of academic skills (e.g., reading, money management), are impaired. There is a somewhat concrete approach to problems and solutions compared with age mates (APA, 2012:34).

Social Domain

Compared with typically developing age mates, the individual is immature in social interactions. For example, there may be difficulty in accurately perceiving peers' social cues. Communication, conversation and language are more concrete or immature than expected for their age. There may be difficulties regulating emotion and behaviours in an age-appropriate fashion; these difficulties are noticed by peers in social situations. There is a limited understanding of risk in social situations, social judgment is immature for their age and the person is at risk of being manipulated by others (gullibility) (APA, 2012:34).

Practical Domain

The individual may function age appropriately in personal care. Individuals may need some support with complex daily living tasks in comparison to peers. In adulthood, supports typically involve grocery shopping, transportation, home and child care organising, nutritious food preparation and banking and money management. Recreational skills resemble those of age mates, although judgment related to the well-being and organisation around recreation requires support. In adulthood, competitive employment is often seen in jobs that do not emphasize conceptual skills. Individuals generally need support to make health-care decisions and legal decisions and to learn to perform a skilled vocation competently. Support is typically needed to raise a family (APA, 2012: 34).

Severity of ID (Moderate Grade)

Conceptual Domain

All through development, the individual's conceptual skills lag markedly behind those peers. For preschoolers, language and pre-academic skills develop slowly. For school-age children, progress in reading, writing mathematics and understanding of time and money occurs slowly across the school years and is markedly limited compared with that of peers. For adults, academic skill development is typically at an elementary level, and support is required for all use of academic skills in work and in personal life. Ongoing assistance on a daily basis is needed to complete conceptual tasks of day-to-day life, and others may take over these responsibilities fully for the individual (APA, 2012:35).

Social Domain

The individual shows marked differences from peers in social and communicative behaviour across development. Spoken language is typically a primary tool for social communication but is much less complex than of peers. Capacity for relationship is evident in ties to family and friends, and the individual may have successful friendships across life and sometimes romantic relations in adulthood.

However, individuals may not perceive or interpret social cues accurately. Social judgment and decision-making abilities are limited, and caretakers must assist the person with life decisions. Friendships with typically developing peers are often affected by communication for social limitation. Significant social and communicative support is needed in work settings for success (APA, 2012:35).

Practical Domain

The individual can care for personal needs involving eating, dressing, elimination and hygiene as an adult, although an extended period of teaching and time is needed for the individual to become independent in these areas, and reminders may be needed. Similarly, participation in all household tasks can be achieved by adulthood, although an extended period of teaching is needed, and ongoing supports will typically occur for adult-level performance.

Independent employment in jobs that require limited conceptual and communication skills can be achieved, but considerable support from co-workers, supervisors and others is needed to manage social expectations, job complexities and ancillary responsibilities, such as scheduling, transportation, health beliefs and money management. A variety of recreational skills can be developed. These typically require additional supports and learning opportunities over an extended period of time. Maladaptive behaviours present in a significant minority causes social problems (APA, 2012:35).

Severity of ID (Severe Grade)

Conceptual Domain

Attainment of conceptual skills is limited. The individual generally has little understanding of written language or of concepts involving numbers, quantity, time and money. Caretakers provide extensive support for problem-solving throughout life (APA, 2012:36).

Social Domain

Spoken language is quite limited in terms of vocabulary and grammar. Speech may be single words or phrases and may be supplemented through argumentative means. Speech and communication are focused on the here and now within everyday events. Language is used for social communication more than for explication. Individuals understand simple speech and general communications. Relationships with family members and familiar others are a source of pleasure and help (APA, 2012:36).

Practical Domain

The individual requires support for all activities of daily living, including meals, dressing, bathing and elimination. The individual requires supervision at all times. The individual cannot make responsible decisions regarding the well-being of self or others. In adulthood, participation in tasks at home, recreational and work requires ongoing support and assistance. Skill acquisition in all domains involves long-term teaching and ongoing support. Maladaptive behaviour, including self-injury, is present at a significant minority (APA, 2012:36).

Severity of ID (Profound Grade)

Conceptual Domain

Conceptual skills generally involve the physical world rather than symbolic processes. The individual may use objects in goal-directed fashion of self-care, work and recreation. Certain visuospatial skills, such as matching and sorting based on physical characteristics, may be acquired. However, co-occurring motor and sensory impairments may prevent functional use of objects (APA, 2012:36).

Social Domain

The individual has very limited understanding of symbolic communication in speech or gesture. He or she may understand some simple instruction or gestures. The individual expresses his/her own desires and emotions largely through nonverbal, non-symbolic communication. The individual enjoys relationships with well-known family members, caretakers and familiar others and initiates and responds to social interactions through gestural and emotional cues. Co-occurring sensory and physical impairments may prevent many social activities (APA, 2012:36).

Practical Domain

The individual is independent on others for all aspects of daily physical care, health and safety, although he or she may able to participate in some of these activities as well. Individuals without severe physical impairments may assist with some daily work tasks at home, like carrying dishes to the table. Simple actions with objects may be the basis of participation in some vocational activities with high levels of ongoing support. Recreational activities may involve, for example, enjoyment in listening to music, watching movies, going out for walks or participating in water activities, all with the support of others. Co-occurring physical and sensory impairments are frequent barriers to participation (beyond watching) in home, recreational and vocational activities. Maladaptive behaviour is present in a significant minority (APA, 2012:36).

COMMUNICATION: A BRIEF OVERVIEW

Communication is crucial in everyday life and in the interaction among individuals. Communication is defined as, from Latin *commūnicāre*, meaning 'to share' and is the act of conveying intended meanings from one entity or group to another through the use of mutually understood signs and semiotic rules (Douglas, 2013). Shannon (2017) affirmed that the main steps inherent to all communication are as follows:

1. The formation of communicative motivation or reason;
2. Message composition (further internal or technical elaboration on what exactly to express);

3. Message encoding (for example, into digital data, written text, speech, pictures gestures and so on);
4. Transmission of the encoded message as a sequence of signals using a specific channel or medium;
5. Noise sources such as natural forces and in some cases human activity (both intentional and accidental) begin influencing the quality of signals propagating from the sender to one or more receivers;
6. Reception of signals and reassembling of the encoded message from a sequence of received signals;
7. Decoding of the reassembled encoded message; and
8. Interpretation and making sense of the presumed original message. (Shannon, 2017: 23-6)

Different Types of Communication

There are different types of communication such as verbal and non-verbal communication, written or non-written communication and interpersonal communication. According to the degree of exchange and involvement of related parties, communication may have the following eight types. Type 1 is the shallowest one, and Type 8 has two ways of mutual involvement and should be the deepest one.

1. Information giving (merely one way not in need of active response).
2. Formal order giving: Authority figure giving orders to subordinate, one way, follow orders, no interpretation and no response. Those with authority can have high emotional input. Those without needs to suppress their emotion.
3. Formal discussion: Two-way communication but highly structural and topics focus on response and interpretation, low emotion sharing.

4. Informal discussion: Two-way communication, low structural and multitopic focus, low emotion sharing.
5. Informal sharing: High and fluent two-way communication, nonstructural, shifting from one topic to another, high emotion sharing. Rational interpretation is replaced by deep emotional sharing.
6. Social Interaction: Continuous informal sharing with high spontaneity and flexibility in response stimuli. Interpretation is highly personal and subjective.
7. One-way involvement: Highly egocentric, one way and personal without any attention outside.
8. Two way involvement and intimacy: Deep emotional sharing, low rationality, interpretation is based on mutual sharing and manifestation of love, hope and trust.

Components in Communication

Among interpersonal communication, there should include the following components such as:

A. Actors (clients, parents, workers, caregivers, significant others, members in the community)
B. Stimuli
C. Media
D. Interpretation
E. Response
F. Use of verbal clues (spoken language, words, syntax)
G. Use of non-verbal clues (gestures, eye contact)
H. Smooth, Blocked,
I. Selectivity and distortion
J. One way, two way
K. Formal vs. informal

L. Information giving, sharing emotion and interest, interaction, involvement.

COMMUNICATION IN PEOPLE WITH INTELLECTUAL DISABILITIES

Communication Problems in People with Intellectual Disabilities

According to the diagnostic criteria of intellectual disability, it is clear the deficits of intellectual function can affect communication and the emotionality of people with intellectual disabilities, and the effects can be in many ways. It can affect the receptibility and understanding of the meaning of others' dialogue in communication and interaction. People with intellectual disabilities may have language problems in understanding the explicit and implicit meanings of various words and sounds. It can affect the spontaneity and flow in communication, expression and sharing of emotion. They may not have enough wording or language ability to do so. The deficit of adaptive ability may make them have poor adjustment to new or unfamiliar environments. Comparing with people with normal intelligence, they may need extra support, understanding, tolerance and patience in helping them in communication and emotional exchange, in particular in meeting unfamiliar people in unfamiliar social and physical environments.

Most people with intellectual disabilities, even at the mild or moderate end of the spectrum, will have some difficulty with communication. This can include any one or a combination of the following (Iacono and Johnson, 2004):

- Speech that is difficult to understand,
- Problems in understanding what is said, or
- Problems in expressing themselves because of limited vocabulary and sentence formulation skills.

In clinical practice, communication problems of people with intellectual disabilities can be summed up as follows:

1. Because of limited intelligence, clients with intellectual disabilities may have limited spoken language to express their ideas or have limited understanding and interpretation of abstract ideas and thinking in communication, in particular those with moderate, severe and profound intellectual disabilities;
2. They are more inclined to use non-verbal clues, such as gestures, eye contact, sound or other means, to express their ideas and emotions. Many of them need visual or audio aids to assist their reception and expression in communication and social interaction;
3. Even in using spoken language, verbal communication may be highly limited. They are inclined to use simple words or use highly symbolic ways to express their ideas and emotions;
4. The use of non-verbal clues, limited spoken language or symbolic use of related clues can be highly specific and unique for individual clients with intellectual disabilities;
5. For deep emotion, in particular those negative ones within intimacy and two-way involvement, clients with intellectual disabilities may use self-harm, aggression, disturbing behaviours and emotional fluctuation (SADE). In some cases, SADE may turn into an obsessive and unconscious mode.
6. There are many types of different communications among different types of actors (clients with clients, clients with caregivers, clients with members in the community, clients with family caregivers). Different pairings of actors may imply different types of communication and different attitudes towards clients' use of related clues; and
7. For clients with intellectual disabilities, their communication may be highly various in different social contexts and environments. They are accustomed to having better communication in a familiar social context as well as those actors who are familiar with them.

A Snapshot of Fluent Communication with People with Intellectual Disabilities

For caregivers in communication with clients with intellectual disabilities, they need to be highly specific, accepting, tolerating and empathic. Tuffrey-Wijine and McEnhill (2008) affirmed effective communication with people with intellectual disabilities should be using simple language, repeated message, enough space, time and understanding. In clinical practice, the following points should be made aware of in fluent communication and interaction with clients with intellectual disabilities:

1. In most cases, they are egocentric and pushy trying to express their egocentric needs in a direct and repeated ways:
2. They have a lack of sufficient wording and language to fully express their needs and emotions;
3. Thus, they tend to express this in a highly symbolic and repeated wording, behaviour and even rituals;
4. Without appropriate understanding of this, workers may even label all these as disturbing behaviours, or challenging behaviours, that demand control and management;
5. Workers need to embrace extra tolerance, patience, acceptance, space and time in understanding the meaning and searching the accurate and appropriate ways in communicating with people with intellectual disabilities;
6. Workers need to go into the context, client's background and emotions behind all these disturbing but highly symbolic expressions;
7. We need to find out the hidden meaning, functions, emotions and needs;
8. We need to connect with clients and fulfill their unexpressed emotions and needs;
9. By doing so, we can interact and communicate with clients with intellectual disabilities smoothly;

10. Even within the behavioural management frame, there should be a baseline context and process to make the behaviour meaningful;
11. In actual practice, an intrinsic reward is much more powerful than an extrinsic one;
12. Intrinsic rewards are actually attachment, holding and caring; and
13. In other words, in interaction with clients with ID, relationship is far more important than control and management.

COMMUNICATION AND SADE: INTERPRETATION AND INTERVENTION

SADE and Communication Problems

As previously mentioned, because of limited intelligence, clients embrace difficulties or even impairments in social interaction. That means, they may have communication problems in daily life and interaction with others. On one hand, they embrace expression hunger to communicate their own views and thinking. On the other hand, they have problems in understanding others' wording and dialogues. In addition, caregivers, because of prolonged overloading caregiving duties and responsibilities, may not enough tolerance, patience and acceptance in understanding the clients with intellectual disabilities. They can always have miscommunication problems between clients and their caregivers. In some cases, miscommunication problems can lead to the occurrence of SADE.

In clinical practice, there are several miscommunication problems that lead to the occurrence of SADE.

Firstly, the clients with intellectual disabilities do not have enough communication abilities, in particular language skills, to express their urgent needs. For example, A is a client with moderate intellectual disability. He is a strong and fat man at around 120 kg body weight. He is impulsive and accustomed to using physical force to resolve difficulties and problems in life. Once, he had a strong need to go to toilet because he drank too much water. While he was rushing to the toilet, a worker who was a slim, short lady weighing only 50 kg blocked his way. Since he did not have enough verbal ability and language skills to voice out his need immediately, he pushed the worker out of his way. Certainly, the slim worker was knocked down and hurt her leg and head. Instead of identifying this as a communication problem, related workers easily labelled A as having aggression and violence. If the worker was hurt seriously or this type of communication problem occurred again in other issues and context, A's aggression and violence inclination would be stereotyped. He would properly be threatened, restrained and isolated by workers. He would also be forced to take antipsychotic medication to decrease his aggression and violent acts.

Secondly, related workers may not have enough experience, tolerance, patience and acceptance to understand the need of clients with intellectual disabilities. The unique but highly repeated and disturbing ways of communication patterns used by the clients may be easily labelled as SADE. For instance, B was a male client with severe intellectual disability. He did not have enough language ability to express his daily life. He had been living in the hostel for ten years already. When he first entered the hostel, he depended on a number of workers to serve his usual need. A worker, Rose, brought him out to have a walk in the community. Another worker, Tom, helped him to go to the toilet. One worker called Mary accompanied him to lunch. One more worker named Richard helped him to return home for home leave. These four workers served him for more than one year. B was quite attached to them. Later, all of them were transferred to other service units. However, B was accustomed to present his needs in names of various workers. Whenever he used the name 'Tom', he presented his need to go to the toilet. Whenever he wanted to go out for lunch, he yelled out the name 'Mary'. When he wanted to return home, then he would say the name 'Richard'. If he wanted to go out, he would say the name 'Rose'. Once, a new worker Jack took care of him. But he did not understand B's unique way of communication. He regarded B's repeated sayings of the names 'Tom' and 'Mary' as disturbing behaviours. The more Jack neglected B's need to go to the toilet and go out, the more

B was annoyed and irritated. Finally, B was furious, he pushed Jack and went out the hostel and urinated near the door. Then B ran away and wandering around the neighborhood. Finally, Jack had to report to the police to find B. From that time onward, Jack was labelled as having aggression and indecent behaviour.

Thirdly, there are spontaneous communication problems between caregivers and clients with intellectual disabilities. This can be a mutually labelling process. The client thinks that the caregiver is bad or rejecting. The worker labels the client as troublemaking or manipulative. They may fixate on an unhappy experience in encountering others. For example, the client may fixate on the memory of being restrained or humiliated by the worker. The worker may also fixate on the memory of the client's aggressive behaviour towards him by pulling her hair suddenly. They do not have enough space, initiative, readiness or opportunities, as well as ability to communicate their emotions and fixation towards one another. As a result, the client becomes more and more aggressive, and the worker becomes more and more authoritarian and labelling.

Related Interventions

Apart from these three situations, communication difficulties are always on the surface of inner deep-seated problems in life, such as unhappy experiences in inmate relationships with significant others or even sufferings and traumas in current or early life. The deeper all these developmental problems and difficulties are, the more complicated and hindering the communication becomes.

Thus, psychosocial interventions in clients with SADE originates from communication difficulties and should be included in the following procedures:

1. Go into the fine details of individuals with SADE in terms of behaviour in context (intensity, frequency, duration, related persons, issues, events, contents, process and details).

2. Understand clients' unfulfilled needs, emotions, cognition, meaning and purpose underlying individual SADE in terms of person in context.
3. If SADE is merely based on communication rather than based on intimacy and trauma, related causes can be discovered in Level 1: behaviours in context interpretation. Related emotions can be discovered Level 2: person in context interpretation. If it is due to intimacy and trauma, then related causes can only be understood in Levels 3, 4 and 5 interpretation.
4. Try to figure out related causes in Level 1 and Level 2. How SADE is influenced by related communication problems. Are these problems only related to certain people, events or issues, as well as physical and social context?
5. In most cases, communication problem-led SADE is incidental and context related. That means, related intervention should focus on improving communication between related people in certain social and physical contexts.
6. Strategies in improving communication should be focussed on three aspects. Firstly, in what ways, clients' communication competence, in particular language skills, receptive ability, response and expression, can be facilitated and changed. Secondly, related workers should enhance their tolerance, acceptance and patience in communication and interaction with the clients with SADE. Thirdly, explore any misunderstandings and miscommunication between related workers and clients and try to resolve them in constructive and meaningful ways for both clients and workers.

All these can be illustrated in, the previously mentioned, A's situation. Because A was labelled as violent and aggressive and had hurt related workers several times, he was forced to take antipsychotic medication. The writer was a professional consultant in this agency. In Level 1 behaviour in context interpretation, A's aggressive behaviour was highly contextual. These aggressive behaviours were intense but low in frequency and short in duration. It all happened within quite a congested physical environment in which a number of persons, including workers and other clients, blocked his way. Also, all these aggressive behaviours happened when he rushed to some place, including the toilet for urination, kitchen for drinking water and getting his favourite sweets from one worker. In addition, he was a client with a severe intellectual disability in which he had limited words and language ability. Furthermore, all this happened to two workers who were slim females. These two workers were young and untrained. They did not know A well and were a bit threatened by A's sudden impulsive running. All this showed that it was merely a communication problem. Based on this interpretation, the following psychosocial interventions were implemented:

1. Educate A to express his needs by facilitating him to speak simple words on going to the toilet, drinking water and sweets. Various kinds of language tools are used in the teaching process.
2. Facilitate related workers to understand, to accept and to be patient with A's aggressive behaviours and communication problems.
3. Enable related workers to learn to how to educate A to express his needs and emotions in an appropriate way, in particular, in urgent situations.
4. Facilitate A to release his physical energy by healthy vigorous exercises such as running and playing ball games.
5. Enable A to beware of the harmful consequences of his impulsive behaviours and to develop appropriate self-control mechanisms.

A Brief Overview on Emotionality

It is based on the book *Emotionality and Mental Illness: A Multi-Dimensional Model* (Yip, 2012). The writer tries to outline an initial conceptual frame on emotionality about primary and secondary emotion, positive and negative emotion, as well as complexity of emotionality in terms of mood, affect, sense and feelings.

It facilitates the readers to have an initial understanding of comprehensive discussion on later chapters in describing blunt affect of schizophrenia, angry feelings of depression, dissociative sense of fear in post-traumatic stress disorder and fluctuating moods in persons with borderline personality disorder.

Rationality and Emotionality

Emotionality is entirely different from rationality. It is entirely misleading to use rational terms to explain human emotion. Furthermore, it is also distorting to regard emotionality as entirely oppositive to rationality. A mentally healthy person can both be affective to others' needs as well as making rational decisions in helping others.

As an opposite, a person with chronic schizophrenia can have blunt affect and irrational response to others. In other words, rationality and emotionality can exist in a parallel form. Following this line of thinking, there should be four combinations of rationality and emotionality. They are listed as follows:

1. Being rational and being emotional/affective;
2. Being irrational and being emotional/affective;
3. Being rational and being apathetic; and
4. Being irrational and being apathetic.

A mature and sensible adult in seeing a beggar in the street can both be rational and affective. S/he is affective to the poor beggar and can be generous enough to give some money to the beggar. But s/he is also rational and aware that the beggar is a stranger to him/her. Thus, s/he would not give too much money and does not allow the beggar to follow him/her. S/he can be irrational and apathetic. S/he does not give any money to the beggar and curses the beggar as lazy and useless.

Logo and Experiences in Emotionality

In fact, in rationality, one looks for logic. In emotionality, one looks for logo (meaning in life). Logic is an art of reasoning. It is a kind of rational explanation of things, no matter if positive or negative things happen.

Emotionality relates to experiences and meaning. In times of severe sufferings, negative emotions such as loneliness, helplessness, inferiority and sadness, as well as hopelessness, happen together. It should be a painful and intolerable experience for the individual. S/he tries hard to make meaning (logo) out of his/her suffering experiences. If s/he cannot make a proper meaning out of it, s/he would intend to end his/her meaningless, painful and intolerable life by committing suicide. However, if s/he can make deep meaning out of his/her sufferings, s/he may develop strong resilience in enduring the sufferings so as to actualise and manifest his/her deep meaning in life.

The deeper the meaning and more worthwhile are the sufferings, the more powerful the resilience in enduring the suffering. Meaning is entirely different from logical explanation. Even if one knows the causes and logic in his/her sufferings. S/he is unable to get rid of the painful feelings and experiences in his/her sufferings.

However, if his/her suffering is highly meaningful, his/her endurance in suffering increases accordingly. For example, a brave soldier is ready to sacrifice his life in a risky mission so as to break the defence line of the enemies. If his mission can be fully accomplished, the whole army will win the battle. In the whole process, s/he can be severely wounded or even lose his/her own life.

But if he can accomplish his mission, he will think that his wounds and suffering are highly worthwhile. Thus, he tries his best to endure the pain and his wounds. Even if he dies, his will power may push him to be alive temporarily until his mission is accomplished.

The Four Components of Emotionality: Feeling, Mood, Affect and Sense

As emotionality is highly dynamic, it involves exchange and interaction among actors. On one hand, it involves internalising emotion from the external environment. On the other hand, it contains externalising deep-seated emotions from the individual. Regarding actors, there are also two major ones: (1) the individual (self) or persons, and (2) object and issues in the external environment (others). According to Yip (2012), there are four major components in emotionality. They are listed as follows:

1. Internalised emotions from external to internal and the focus is on self (feeling);
2. Externalised emotions from internal to external and the focus is on self (mood);
3. Internalise emotions from external to internal and the focus is on others (sense); and
4. Externalised emotions from internal to external and the focus is on others (affect).

These four components interact and intermingle with one another forming the dynamic emotionality in the day-to-day emotional exchange within and among every individual. Each of them has their own complexity and nature. According to Yip (2012), feeling involves many layers. There are the feelings of: Layer 1, immediate social and physical environment; Layer 2, recent period of time; Layer 3, life pattern and hobbies; Layer 4, selfhood and personality; and Layer 5, ontological sense of existence. Feelings in various layers moves along. It can be vertical movement up and down among various layers. It can also be horizontal movement in a single layer among different issues, objects and persons. It can be maximizing refined details in one issue, person or object. Or it can be minimizing or being away from one object, issue and person. Mood can have a different intensity, duration and frequency. The deeper the feeling is internalised, the more intensive and durable the mood is externalised. The shallower the feeling is internalised, the easier the mood is externalised. Affect can be an immediate response to other emotions or can be a delayed response. Affect can exist in various defence mechanisms, such as projection, sublimation, denial, regression, introjection, fantasy, repression and suppression. Sense is spontaneous perception of the external environment. It can be sense of mind, sense of body, sense of self, sense of environment, sense of growth and sense of being.

These four dynamic components intermingle with one another. For example, the deeper the feeling is internalised, the more intensive the mood is externalised. Within a traumatic experiences, the individual experiences traumatic senses of self, body, mind and environment. Such traumatic senses are firmly anchored in the individual's memories and becomes deeply internalised feelings. They may last for life.

Primary Negative Emotions

Emotions can be primary and secondary. Primary emotion means that related emotion is primary and cannot be further reduced. Secondary emotion means that related emotion is combined by several or more than one emotion. For negative emotions, related studies and clinical practice show that there are five primary emotions. They are inferiority, fear, anger, loneliness and emptiness.

Regarding inferiority, it is a kind of primary negative emotion when one feels incompetent or unable to achieve or accomplish certain tasks. Or it can be a sense of inadequacy in comparing with others. Sometimes it turns to a kind of poor self-image thinking that one is much poorer than others in most aspects of life. In a positive sense, inferiority can be a driving force, pushing one to learn from others, to be humble in front of authority figures and a supernatural phenomenon or even God. In terms of emotionality, inferiority can also exist in forms of feeling, mood, affect and sense.

Fear is a primary emotion helping one to keep away or to avoid danger and risky situations so as to protect one from being hurt. Fear can be anticipated and gradually aroused when one is approaching dangerous situation, or it can be aroused when danger and attacks come suddenly. Intensive fear can hinder one's courage and determination to do certain things, to encounter certain persons and to go to certain places. In terms of emotionality, fear can also present in forms of feeling, mood, affect and sense.

Anger is an explosive primary emotion preparing one to face and deal with danger, conflict and confrontation directly and squarely. It arouses one's deep-seated drive of aggression and extinction of opponents and enemies. In positive terms, it gives us extra courage as well as psychic and mental energy to counteract attack, defend ourselves and prepare us mentally and physically for defence, fight and attack. In terms of emotionality, anger can also manifest in forms of affect, feeling, mood, and sense.

Loneliness is a primitive emotion driving one to be together with others within a family, social and community circle. It encourages us to interact, to relate and to connect with others. As the human is a kind of social animal, the feeling of loneliness is particularly strong when one is not being accepted or included in his/her social circle. It manifests in forms of affect, sense, mood and feeling.

Emptiness is a primary emotion originated from a primitive drive to explore, to discover and to be involved in certain meaningful activities in everyday life. It enables us to be involved in cultural activities and creation. It facilitates us to search and anchor our meaning of life. When such meaningful activities and involvements cease, one can feel empty, bored and meaningless.

Chronic emptiness means that one has lost his/her meaning of life. In terms of emotionality, it can exist in forms of feeling, mood, affect and sense. Each of these five primitive emotions may mean different manifestations in feeling, mood, affect and sense. They can be illustrated in the following table.

Table. Presentation of Feeling, Mood, Affect and Sense in Five Primary Emotions

	Content of Feeling	Related Affect	Related Mood	Related Sense
Inferiority	I am not competent Others are better than me I am useless No matter how hard I try, still I am not OK	Seeing, admiring others strengths and positivity Thinking that others can attain without trying hard or failure likes me Others will look down upon me	Down and unstable in facing others Up but unstable when facing others' appreciation Hyposensitive mood in response to others' comment especially negative ones Subtle, long duration and frequent when facing others' negative comment	Crying and mourning Strong sense of inferiority may turn to withdrawal from social activities Unable to fulfill external demand and request
Fear	I am afraid I want to avoid danger It is dangerous, fearful, I have to stay away from it	They hate me They want to hurt me They are horrible, unmanageable and uncontrollable	Intensive mood when facing fearful objects Residual fear even when keeping away from feared object Acute and intensive when facing fearful objects Subtle but long duration when being away from fearful objects	Screaming and hysterical, sometimes fight back Strong and unavoidable fear may make one feel depersonalised and dissociative from self and reality
Anger	I am angry I have tolerated enough	Others are bad ones They deserve suffering and punishment	Explosive and intensive during anger explosion Released mood and sense of self-satisfaction when anger is exploded to related target	Sense of powerfulness Sense of capability

Table (Continued)

	Content of Feeling	Related Affect	Related Mood	Related Sense
Anger	You are too much Anger can turn inwards in forms of self-hate	They have to be hurt, bullied and extinguished	Very strong, intense and explosive during fight back Released and cool down when anger is properly channeled and the object is destructed by anger	Expanded sense of mastery control Decreased response to possible risks and harm Unsettled stimuli and disturbed harmony of mind and body
Loneliness	I am lonely No one cares about me No one understands me	Others are apathetic and careless Others are keeping a distance from me Others do not respond to my feeling or behaviour	Nervous and tense when together with others Down and subtle when away from others Urge to be attached and dependent on others. Unhappy and frustrated when faced with separation	Decreased satisfaction in daily activities if such activities are performed alone Retarded response to external stimuli and demand Overreactive or agitated in facing being together with others
Emptiness	Life is so boring It is meaningless Nothing can be done and nothing should be done	Apathetic to external events Life and struggle by me and by others are meaningless What people perform is aimless and purposeless Blunt affect to external stimuli	Stagnant and sinking mood in forms of internal vacuum Long duration and endless internal deadness	Slow psychomotor response or simple no motion Lack of motivation to commit any activities or achieve anything

Primary and Secondary Negative Emotions

Secondary negative emotions are combinations of two or more than two negative emotions. For example, sadness is a combination of loneliness and inferiority. Envy is a combination of inferiority, fear and anger. When A is envious of B, A feels inferior in front of B. It is because B, in a certain area, is much better than A. Together with this is that A is afraid, sooner or later, B will take over him/her. In doing so, A may finally lose his/her own social status, benefits and advantages. In addition to that, A is also angry with B. That means envy is actually a combination of fear, anger and inferiority. However, the sense of inferiority is deep-seated and covered by anger and fear. Similarly, hate is a combination of anger and fear. In normal circumstances in which anger can be aired out easily towards the opponent in the social environment, hate cannot be formulated. However, if the individual harbours fear, hate can be formulated. For instance, in an office setting, C is humiliated by his oppressive boss. As this job is very important for C, he cannot air out his anger towards his boss. His deep-seated fear of losing his job inhibits the airing out of anger. The more it is inhibited, the more hateful feelings are developed and restored within the individual. The internalised feeling of hate, once being stored up, may gradually accumulate to an intolerable level. Sooner or later, the deep-seated and accumulated hateful feelings may externalise in forms of intensive aggression, revenge and attack. Thus, for psychosocial interventions for persons with secondary negative emotions, it is important to reflect different sorts of primary negative emotions consisting within the secondary emotions. For instance, if C seeks counselling from a social worker in a counselling centre, related social workers need to acknowledge and reflect C's fear towards his oppressive boss. Once this fear is ventilated, his anger can gradually elaborate and communicate. Below are some common complicated secondary emotions and their related components.

1. Sadness = inferiority + loneliness + helplessness (an individual female feels sad about the death of her husband because s/he feels

dreadfully lonely and helpless after the death of the husband. In addition to that, she also feels inferior and being abandoned by her deceased husband).

2. Anxiety = fear + helplessness and inferiority (an individual being kept within an intensive anxiety always feels that s/he fails to meet the demand of his/her significant other. S/he contains fear and worries that if s/he fails to meet such a demand, sooner or later, s/he may lose the love, acceptance and permission of his/her significant other. His/her sense of inferiority may thus be provoked. To ease out all these unpleasant emotions, s/he asks for others' help. If no one can offer help, his/her sense of helplessness prevails. Finally, her/his fear and anxiety level may reach an intolerable level. Thus, s/he manifests these negative emotions in various forms of anxiety disorders with both somatic and emotional symptoms.

Primary and Secondary Positive Emotions

Human beings do not survive on negative emotions; instead, they strive for positive emotions. With each primary negative emotion, there are corresponding positive emotions. In fact, positive emotions and negative emotions exist together. With prevailing fear, individuals look for security and protection. Within overwhelming inferiority, individuals aspire for self-confidence and senses of superiority. In loneliness, individuals urge for the togetherness of other persons. For persons with intense anger, they feel deeply humiliated, rejected or isolated. Thus, deep down in their mind, they still look for love, caring and genuine acceptance. Similarly, deep down in ontological emptiness, an individual still hopes that sooner or later, s/he can live a life with full meaningfulness and substantiality.

A deep look on positive emotions such as security, self-confidence, togetherness, acceptance, substantiality and meaningfulness reviews that all these positive emotions rest upon the fundamental positive natures of human nature. There are love, hope and trust. Everyone aspires for love and being loved, hope and being hopeful, as well as trust and being trustful. For example, an individual who grows up in a family with love, hope and trust certainly feels secure, confident, accepting and substantial in life. As an opposite, an individual who grows up in a family without love, hope and trust certainly feels anxious, insecure, fearful, inferior, lonely, angry and empty in life.

Regarding love, hope and trust, they are, in fact, basic ingredients in formulating intimate bonding for an individual. However, in day-to-day social interaction, an individual can have several levels in relating to others with love, hope and trust. They are touch, encounter, and bonding. 'Touch' means that in a casual interaction with a certain person, the individual suddenly feels being loved or love, being hopeful or hope, as well as being trustful and trust. It impresses the individual, but it comes and goes. It is just like when you suddenly fall down on a stairway, a kind-hearted person holds your hand and helps you stand firm to avoid falling. You are so grateful for his/her help that you feel their concern and being cared for. 'Encounter' means that the individual, after a constant and regular interaction with a friend, a colleague or a peer, finally finds that s/he encounters a good person with love, hope and trust in relating to this person. 'Bonding' means that the individual has a constant, regular and intimate relationship with his/her significant other with love, hope and trust.

Certainly, 'bonding', in particular with significant others, is crucial for the maturity, survival and meaning of life for every human being. Within a good affective bonding, such as parent-child bonding and husband-wife bonding, concerned members have three characteristics. The first one is that members are willing to sacrifice for one another. An affective mother, because of deep love, has hope and trust towards her son, and she is willing to donate her kidney to her son who has kidney failure. The second characteristic is that members share common beliefs, values, thinking and deeds. It is common to observe that a son walks, talks and behaves similar to his father. The final one is that they urge the presence of one another in facing happiness, hardship, difficulties and attainment in life. The presence of others with deep bonding makes the individual feel more complete and actualised. For example, in a graduation ceremony, a son properly feels more complete with the presence of his parents.

Unresolved Emotional Complexes

Emotionality is complicated and dynamic. In actual life, a person with intense inferiority may hide his/her inferiority within a deep concealment of superiority. Within social interaction, s/he grasps every chance to prove that s/he is competent, elegant and superior. S/he even needs to exploit, oppress and humiliate others to sustain his/her sense of superiority. In that occasion, s/he is kept within a superior and inferior complex. Similarly, a person with a prevailing sense of fear tries his/her best to avoid seeing anything or any person who triggers his/her sense of fear. The fear and avoidance complex may go on until his/her fear towards this person, object or thing is finally resolved. However, if the fearful person is someone s/he deeply loves in life, s/he engages in an approach and avoidance complex. On one hand, s/he aspires to connect and interact with this person so as to feel warm and being loved. On the other hand, s/he is afraid, in encountering with this person, and s/he may be humiliated, oppressed and abused again. That means, together with the approach and avoidance complex, s/he also harbours a love and hate complex towards this person. In the same way, a person with overwhelming sense of ontological emptiness and boredom may try his/her best to fill up his/her inner vacuum by an unhealthy addiction, such as substance abuse, compulsive gambling and/or sex addiction. In other words, within five primary negative emotions. They are five corresponding unresolved emotional complexes. They can be listed as follows:

1. Inferiority (superiority and inferiority complex);
2. Fear (fear and avoidance complex or approach and avoidance complex);
3. Anger (love and hate complex);
4. Loneliness (loneliness and togetherness complex); and

5. Emptiness (emptiness and obsession complex).

All these emotional complexes complicate the process of expression, communication, interaction and manifestation of emotionality. In actual practice, related professionals should be sensitive and competent enough to recognise, to interact and to resolve all these complexes in clients' emotionalities.

Interaction and Mutual Influence among Negative Emotions

In actual clinical practice, apart from acknowledging clients' unresolved emotional complexes, clients' negative emotions intermingle and mutually influence one another. There are several levels of mutual influence among negative emotions. They are listed as follows:

Level 1: Emotional Complexes (inferiority and superiority complex; loneliness and togetherness complex; love and hate complex; approach and avoidance complex; emptiness and addiction complex).

Level 2: Horizontal Mutual Influence (fear and anger are mutually inhibiting; loneliness and inferiority are mutually inhibiting).

Level 3: Vertical Mutual Influence (inferiority and fear are mutually reinforcing; anger and loneliness are mutually reinforcing).

Level 4: Diagonal Mutual Influence and Complication (inferiority and anger are mutually complicating; loneliness and fear are mutually complicating).

Level 5: Ambivalence of Emotions (a full combination of fear, loneliness, inferiority and anger leading to ontological boredom and emptiness).

In clinical practice, the lower the level of mutual influence among emotions, the easier to communicate and understood. The higher the level is, the more difficult and complicated the mutual influence among emotions.

In Level 2, emotions inhibit one another. For example, with fear, anger cannot be fully expressed. Anger combines with fear to formulate deep-seated hate. As a contrary, deeply inhibited fear needs anger to ventilate out. It is a flight (fear) and fight mechanism that is commonly observed in people with anxiety disorder. Similarly, loneliness and inferiority are inhibited to one another. For example, when one feels lonely, one goes outside and searches for togetherness with friends and peers. However, when s/he gets together with his/her peers, s/he feels inferior in comparing with others. Once the sense of inferiority arouses, s/he properly needs to withdraw from this relationship with others.

In Level 3, inferiority interacts with fear. Similarly, loneliness interacts with anger. They reinforce one another. That means, when inferiority combines with fear, inferiority becomes more intensive and complicated. Also, when fear combines with inferiority, fear becomes more intensive and complicated. For example, when one encounters a car accident, s/he is involved in a deep traumatic fear. At the same time, s/he also feels inferior, as s/he cannot control the occurrence of the car accident.

In Level 4, the situation is even more complicated. That is a diagonal interaction between anger and inferiority, as well as between loneliness and fear. In this level, individual emotional response is complicated and intensive. It certainly makes the individual impulsive and uncontrollable to his/her manifestation of negative emotions. In fact, Level 4 is a combination of Level 2 and Level 3 together. For instance, E is a delinquent adolescent who has a large and odd tattoo over his body. F is a passerby and attends to E's tattoo. Unfortunately, F stares at E in an unfriendly manner. It deeply irritates E. He is furious and prepared to attack E. In that situation, it is clear that E's anger is closely integrated with his senses of fear and inferiority. E feels highly humiliated by F's staring. E also feels fearful of being threatened by F's impolite attitude. That means, E's anger is mixed with inferiority and fear. To resolve this, F needs to provide a sense of security for E (fear and security complex Level 1). In doing so, it is a Level 2 movement in which anger is inhibited by fear. Then E has to ensure that F's sense of superiority is consolidated (inferiority and superiority complex). In doing so, it is a Level 3 movement in which inferiority is related with fear. In resolving the Level 4 emotion, individuals need to go back to emotional movement in Level 2, Level 1 and Level 3.

In Level 5, there is a combination of four primary negative emotions, fear, loneliness, anger and inferiority. When the individual experiences all these primary negative emotions, s/he feels ambivalent, confused and bored. With that ambivalence of four primary emotions, individuals develop emptiness. That means, it is a kind of ontological emptiness with an absence of meaning of life.

Presentation of Emotions

Emotions may not be presented in a direct way by the individuals. It can be presented in an indirect way. In day-to-day emotional communication, there may be the following ways of presentations:

1. Direct presentation (one presents his/her emotion directly)
2. Indirect presentation
   a. Use of paradox (that means, individual uses opposite emotion to cover up his/her real emotion. For instance, if s/he feels inferior, s/he tries to appear as competent and superior)
   b. Use of metaphor (that means, the individual uses various types of metaphors such as storytelling, poem and artwork to represent his/her emotions)
   c. Use of symbol (that means, the individual uses social, cultural and private symbols to present his/her emotions)
   d. Use of rituals (that means, the individual performs certain rituals to present his/her emotion. It can be religious rituals or cultural rituals such as rituals in marriage or funeral)

e. Use of refined details (that means, the individual fixates on mentioning certain refined details in certain persons, events or issues so as to present his/her emotions)
f. Use of repetition (that means, the individual continuously repeats certain details, rituals, metaphor, symbols or behaviours to manifest his/her emotions
g. Missing emotions (that means, the individual does not manifest appropriate emotions. For instance, one appears as a clam and numbed after a traumatic accident
h. Overventilation and overuse of emotions (that means, individual tends to fixate on one type of emotion to present other forms of emotions. For instance, one may use anger to represent concern and care to others)

All these have important implications for clinical interventions with clients with emotional and mental problems. Related professionals should be fully aware of clients' unique ways in presentation their emotions. For direct narration, related professionals should help their clients to recognise, connect and share corresponding layers of feelings, intensity, frequency and duration of mood, types of senses, and defence mechanisms in affect within clients' emotion. For indirect presentation of emotions, related professionals should also connect, express and resolve clients' emotions in indirect ways so that clients feel more at ease and relaxed in emotional connection and ventilation.

SADE and Emotionality in People with Intellectual Disabilities

In comparing with people with normal intelligence, people with intellectual disabilities have some special features in feeling, mood, affect and sense. They have problems in communication and expression of their thinking and emotions.

Feeling: Using Layer 1 and 2 to Express Deep Layers 3, 4 and 5

The deeper the layer of the feeling, the more complicated it is and the more difficult it can be expressed. For clients with intellectual disabilities, they are accustomed to using Layer 1 (feeling of immediate physical and social environment) and Layer 2 (feeling of recent period of time) to replace or substitute Layer 3 (feeling of life pattern and hobbies), Layer 4 (feeling of personality and self system) and Layer 5 (feeling of meaning of life or ontological existence). The more severe their intellectual disability, the shallower their feeling of expression. For example, a client with moderate intellectual disability earnestly waits for the visit of his father. He harbours deep complicated feelings towards his father and his visit; what he can express and interpret is only Layer 1. Thus, he keeps on asking his worker when his father will arrive. The worker simply answers him that his father will arrive around 2:00 p.m. Despite him having answered many times, he keeps on asking once every fifteen minutes. Another experienced worker who knows the client well tries to channel all these feelings in deep layers. When the client asks when his father will arrive, apart from saying the exact time, the worker tries to say, 'Are you looking earnestly for the coming of your father?' The client says, 'Yes'. The worker then says, 'Are you afraid that your father will not come?' The client nods his head. The worker keeps on saying, 'If your father does not come, I will go out together with you and go to the same Chinese restaurant for lunch. OK?' After this affirmation and channeling of the client's deeper layer of feeling of insecurity, uncertainty and loneliness towards his father's visit, the client becomes more stable and his continuous and disturbing asking ceases.

Mood: Difficulties in Appropriate Mood Expression

Because of limited intelligence, clients with intellectual disabilities harbour difficulties and problems in communication and expression of emotion. As mood is a ventilation and expression of various layers of feelings, they have difficulties in appropriate mood expression and ventilation. They may have difficulties in ventilating moods in appropriate intensity, frequency and duration. They may have problems in using appropriate language, word and style of mood ventilation. They have harbour strong expressions of hunger in which they feel anxious and nervous in mood ventilation. All these can turn into SADE. For example, a client with an intellectual disability, when they feel angry with his or her significant other, may not have enough language ability and wording to express his anger. Instead, he may ventilate his/her anger in aggressive acts, such intense hitting, pulling others' hair or destruction of objects. Similarly, an intellectually disabled client with autism feels highly anxious and insecure as his/her parents fail to pick him/her up at the normal scheduled time. Instead of expressing his/her anxiety and fear in appropriate wording and tone, s/he may simply yell in a loud voice and repeat some mild self-harm behaviours.

Affect: Inappropriate Affect Response

Because of their limited intelligence, clients with intellectual disabilities usually have problems in receiving, interpretation and responding to external stimuli. That means, their cognitive and emotional processing may be slower than people with normal intelligence, especially in emotional attunement and deep and implicit emotional exchange. They tend to receive, interpret and respond in a directive and/simple way. For people with normal intelligence, paradox and metaphor may be used. But it may not be understood by people with an intellectual disability. The more severe the intellectual disability, the slower and more difficult the client is in responding to external stimuli and others' emotions. They tend to be more egocentric in expressing their emotions or ventilation of their own mood. In some situations, they may have inappropriate affect responses to others.

Sense: Sense of Body and Desire Driven

Sense is spontaneous reception from external stimuli with a consciousness and sense of existence. There is a sense of body, sense of mind, sense of self and sense of environment. For clients with intellectual disabilities, because of their limited intelligence, their sense of mind and self may be slower and limited in comparison with people with normal intelligence. However, their sense of body may be highly sensitive. That means, they may be more desire driven. They are more inclined to sensatory stimulation and bodily senses. Regarding sense of growth or sense of existence, they are severely affected by intellectual disability. For example, quite a number of intellectually disabled clients with severe autism strive for sensatory stimulation in forms of rocking movement or scratching of a body part. Most clients with intellectual disabilities are fond of sweets and good food as sensatory stimulation.

Negative Emotions in People with Intellectual Disability

Clients with intellectual disabilities are limited in emotional presentation and life exposure; they may have special features in their negative emotions.

Firstly, they are more vulnerable to stress, harm, traumas and abandonment, as well as suffering. They easily embrace various forms of negative emotions, such as loneliness, inferiority, anger and fear. A stressful event for people with normal intelligence may be traumatic for people with intellectual disabilities. The more severe the intellectual disability, the more vulnerable the client becomes. In addition, facing this traumatic event, the client has difficulty in presenting and ventilating all these negative emotions.

Secondly, because of their limited intelligence, their mood container is limited in size; they are less able to rationalise, interpret and contain related negative emotions. Their emotional control mechanism is simple. Their negative emotions can be easily triggered. For example, when their emotional container is overflowing, anger may be triggered and ventilate in two forms. One is projection and another one is displacement. Projection means that the client with the intellectual disability may simply assume all bad things are due to a fixated person. So the client will throw his/her anger in forms of verbal and physical aggression towards this person. Displacement means once the emotional container is full, the client will throw out his/her anger to the nearest people or things immediately.

Thirdly, they may be afraid of external authority figures who inhibit them in expressing all these negative emotions. Their negative emotions may be temporarily suppressed and displaced or impulsively burst out to other persons, in particular their significant others. In some cases, the process can be delayed for several months or years. For example, C is a client with an intellectual disability. He had been repeatedly verbally and physically abused by a worker in a sheltered workshop. However, because of intense fear, he tried to repress all these traumatic experiences and related negative emotions. Finally, he was transferred to a more humanistic vocational rehabilitation service unit in another agency. Related workers were humanistic and caring. All these fixated and repressed traumatic memories and anger were activated. So the client was able to rebounce all these traumatic memories and anger. Thus, he displaced his anger by expressing aggression towards his mother and related workers who cared about him.

Fourthly, very often, all these negative emotions may also be expressed in SADE. That are self-harm (anger turns inward, inferiority), aggression (anger turns outward, fear of loss, inferiority), disturbing behaviour (loneliness, attachment hunger) and emotional fluctuation (mood fluctuation with high intensity, high frequent or long duration).

Fifthly, in some cases, the fear of loss and anger are highly internalised, and clients with intellectual disabilities cannot be expressed clearly. Instead, worries and anxieties are accumulated and manifested. For clients with severe and profound intellectual disabilities, all these worries and anxieties can turn into severe psychosomatic problems, such as constipation or ulcers.

Sixthly, secondary emotions and emotional complexes are less likely to be formulated, in particular those with moderate and severe intellectual disability. Instead, simple and primary negative emotions are easily expressed.

Finally, clinical practice shows that clients with intellectual disabilities are *mostly vulnerable to loneliness* because of dependence in lifelong fatigue of their caregivers. Following this are *abandonment, fear and anger*, as they are frequently transferred from one service unit to another in the life developmental process. Interestingly, only clients with mild or mildly moderate intellectual disability will harbour inferiority, as they have enough intelligence to compare their performance with those people with normal intelligence.

Positive Emotions in People with Intellectual Disabilities

Regarding positive emotions, people with intellectual disabilities may harbour the following characteristics:

1. Similar to a small child, clients with intellectual disabilities can have positive emotions because of simplified id-based desires and satisfaction in having something sweet to eat, going out for meals or hitting others for fun.
2. They can also be happy in companionship with friends as well as expecting parents and family caregivers to visit them in the coming future.
3. However, all these simple desires and wishes need to be fulfilled immediately or else they may feel puzzled and anxious.
4. They have strong attachment needs and dependence on their parents in which their sense of hope and being hopeful, love and being loved, trust and being trusted are closely related to the attitudes and caring of their parents towards them.
5. Nevertheless, because of various reasons (overdemanding, marital discord, divorce, aging, family dynamics), family caregivers/or and parents may have fatigue, be rejecting, emotionally neglecting and manipulating to clients with intellectual disabilities, making their urge for love, hope and trust be in vain.

6. All this deprivation for love, hope and trust may not be properly expressed by clients with intellectual disabilities. Instead, they may express these in forms of self-harm, aggression and disturbing behaviours.
7. Instead of focussing clients' hidden urges for love, hope and trust, related workers may simply focus on behavioural control, medication, restraints, time out or even institutionalisation towards their self-harm, aggression and disturbing behaviours, making their sense of being neglected, abandoned and rejected intensify further.

Presentation of Emotion in People with Intellectual Disabilities

Because of their limited intelligence, their presentation of emotions may have the following features:

1. They may not be able to directly communicate their emotions, views and needs, as they may not have enough language ability, wording and spontaneity as people with normal intelligence.
2. They are inclined to use symbols in communication and presentation of emotions. However, all these symbols may be highly personal and unique to individual clients. Some may use different sounds, simple wording, names of caregivers, gestures, pictures or even SADE to express their emotions.
3. Their deep-seated emotions in facing abandonment, abuse, separation and other unhappy events may be too difficult to express, leading to prolonged suppression and repression with blank emotions and blunt affect.
4. In some cases, all these repressed emotions can accumulate to an extent that leads to sudden outbursts or impulsive expression of self-harm or aggression towards their significant others.
5. For some clients, their memories towards their lost significant others can be expressed in forms of refined and repeat rituals of actions, deeds or wordings.

EMOTIONALITY AND SADE: HUMANISTIC INTERVENTION

Humanistic Intervention Procedures

Facing the previously mentioned SADE because of problems in emotionality, psychosocial interventions should include the following procedures:

1. Go into the fine details with individuals with SADE in terms of behaviour in context (intensity, frequency, duration, related persons, issues, events, contents, process and details).
2. Understand clients' unfulfilled needs, emotions, cognition, meaning and purpose underlying the individual's SADE in terms of person in context.
3. If SADE is merely based on emotionality rather than based on intimacy and trauma, related causes can be discovered in Level 1: behaviours in context interpretation. Related emotions can be discovered Level 2: person in context interpretation. If it is due to intimacy and trauma, then related causes can only be understood in Levels 3, 4 and 5 interpretation.
4. Try to figure out related causes in Level 1 and Level 2. How SADE is influenced by related problems in communication and emotion problems. The client has problems in sharing, ventilation and expression of his/her positive or negative emotions with people, events and issues, as well as physical and social context.
5. In most cases, communication-problem-led SADE is highly patterned and consistent. That means, related intervention should focus on helping the client to share, ventilate and express his/her positive or negative emotions appropriately with related people in certain social and physical contexts.
6. A comprehensive and thorough understanding and interpretation of clients' SADE in relation to their problems in emotionality includes:

a. Using Levels 1 and 2 feelings to express Levels 3, 4 and 5 feelings;
b. Difficulties in appropriate mood expression and ventilation;
c. Poor mood containing and processing;
d. Inappropriate affect response;
e. Desire-driven sense of body to replace sense of mind and sense of self;
f. Vulnerability of stress to become trauma;
g. Loss and anger turn into worries, anxieties and psychosomatic symptoms;
h. Suppressed, unexpressed and repressed emotional complexes (superiority inferiority complex, loneliness and aloneness complex, fear and security complex, approach and avoidance complex, and love and hate complex);
i. Uncontrollable urges in companionship, id-based desires, loneliness and fear of being abandonment;
j. Insufficient language ability, intelligence and skills to present emotion accurately, directly and spontaneously;
k. Highly personal symbolic way in emotional expression, which is only understood by those caring and empathic caregivers and/or significant others;
l. Blank emotion of blunt affect because of prolonged repression and suppression;
m. Sudden impulsive overflowing of negative emotions; and
n. Present emotions in repeated refined fixated rituals.

7. Strategies in improving clients' emotionality should be focused on several aspects. Firstly, facilitate clients to express and ventilate emotions by appropriate wording, gestures, skills and language. Secondly, educate clients' caregivers and significant others to understand, accept and tolerate clients' inappropriate mood expression and ventilation, in particular in forms of SADE. Thirdly, encourage regular and healthy release of clients' negative emotions by constructive and meaningful activities, such as physical

exercise, music, singing, social interaction and recreational activities. All these may be shown in the following case illustration.

Helping Tommy to Express His Emotions and Needs

Tommy was a client with autism and intellectual disability in a day activities centre. Despite Tommy enjoying most activities in this centre, he was highly sensitive and fixated on a rigid time and daily schedule. Every day, his mother took him home at 4:00 p.m. At 3:30 p.m., he refused to do anything and waited for his mother. If his mother was late, he would be highly anxious and engaged, manifesting in frequent head bumping self-harm behaviours. Once, his mother was an hour late because of traffic congestion. Tommy was highly anxious, he cried bitterly and unintentionally bit his worker. Related workers tended to regard all these as autistic features, he was sent to a psychiatrist and antipsychotic medication, antidepressant, and anxiety medication were given. As the writer was the clinical consultant of the agency, related workers were encouraged to undergo behaviour in context and person in context interpretation.

In behaviour in context interpretation, it showed that whenever Tommy felt anxious, he would first stay quiet and be involved in deep thinking for around ten minutes. Then he began to bump his head. It began with slow action and gradually increased in frequency and intensity. Related workers approached him and reminded him to stop this, saying that his mother was coming. However, the more the worker said this, the more intense his head bumping was. After fifteen minutes, if her mother was still not there, he would jump up and down and yell out loudly.

In person in context interpretation, the related workers discussed together and discovered that Tommy harboured an intense intimate need in being together with his mother. One worker disclosed that Tommy's father deserted him when he was only ten years old. His mother was emotionally enmeshed with Tommy. That means, Tommy felt insecure and fear when his mother was late. He might be afraid that his mother was going to abandon him. Within the ten minutes, he remained quiet and involved in deep thinking, and he might recall all the unhappy memories in the past.

He felt sad, unhappy, helpless and his anger towards his father may turn inwards as self-hatred and manifest in forms of head bumping. All these are intolerable and painful for him. That was why he yelled out and jumped up and down to release this self-directed anger.

All this showed that Tommy had problems venting his intense feelings of insecurity, helplessness and self-directed anger. By knowing this, related workers tried to teach Tommy to vent all these by referring to some cards with different facial expressions. In addition to this, Tommy was helped to speak out simple words such as 'I am angry', 'I was sad', I feel upset' or 'I am afraid Mother will abandon me'. When Tommy learnt to voice out all these feelings, his self-harm behaviour gradually decreased. In addition, he was encouraged to join in a jogging team in which his physical energy was released properly.

CONCLUSION

As a conclusion, this chapter is a comprehensive discussion on emotionality and communication of persons with intellectual disabilities and how SADE is related to problems and difficulties in communication and emotionality.

The chapter begins with a description of diagnosis and features of intellectual disability and follows with an overview of communications and emotionality. Then, problems and difficulties of emotionality and communication of people with intellectual disabilities are mentioned. Finally, interpretation and intervention of clients with SADE in terms of emotionality and communication are discussed.

Chapter 4

INTIMACY AND ATTACHMENT OF CLIENTS WITH INTELLECTUAL DISABILITIES: IMPLICATIONS IN INTERPRETATION AND INTERVENTION OF SADE

INTRODUCTION

Chapter four is a comprehensive articulation of intimacy and attachment need of clients with intellectual disabilities. Because of limited intelligence and exposure to opportunities in life, many of them need to depend on caregivers. Comparatively speaking, their intimacy and attachment needs are more intense than people with normal intelligence. However, because of overwhelming caregiving, many family caregivers fail to fulfill clients' intimacy and attachment needs. Some even abandon them or put them in boarding schools or residential care and day care centres, even at a very young age. Many of them stay in these facilities for their whole lives. Home leave or union with their family members becomes a luxury. Most of them earnestly need to have intimate contact with others. They easily regard caregivers in service units as substitute attachment figures. Their attachment hunger easily expresses in forms of disturbing behaviours. However, many workers may regard these as challenging behaviours and try to ignore them. As a consequence, attachment hunger prevails and transforms into self-harm and aggression. This situation is particularly serious for those intellectually disabled clients facing sequential loss of attachment figures. Various intervention strategies in fulfilling clients' intimacy and attachment needs in different service units are also thoroughly discussed.

THE IMPORTANCE OF INTIMACY FOR CLIENTS WITH INTELLECTUAL DISABILITIES

The Importance of Intimacy for Human Beings

Intimacy is crucial for a human being's development. We are social animals. We need to relate to others in the whole life process. When we are young, we need to adhere to our parents. We depend on physical, psychological and social holding from our parents so that we can develop physically, psychologically and socially. In our childhood and adolescence, apart from intimacy with our parents and siblings, we also develop intimate relationships with our classmates, friends and peers. Within these intimate friendships, we develop our social network, learning how to relate to others as well as how to establish social relationships with different groups of people.

In youth and adulthood, on one hand, the need of intimacy is gratified in courtship and marriage. On the other hand, individuals are mature enough to provide intimacy to their partners, children and family members. That means, intimacy is crucial in human beings in terms of the following:

- Intimacy is the main ingredient in the formation of family, courtship and friendship.
- Intimacy facilitates and generates, love and being loved, hope and being hopeful and trust and being trustworthy.

- Intimacy is the breeding bed for human development in infancy, childhood, adolescence, youth, adulthood and aging.

Intimacy is closely related to other human dimensions, such as meaning of life, selfhood, emotionality, morality, embodiment and social functioning. In other words, intimacy is related to:

- Self-identity and development of the self system;
- Gender and sex identity;
- Emotionality;
- Social development and relationship with others;
- Psychological development and cognition;
- Morality; and
- Spirituality and meaning of life.

All these are influenced by intimate relationships with some crucial attachment figures in life.

Intimacy Features for Clients with Intellectual Disabilities

For a client with an intellectual disability, their limited intelligence may imply a greater demand than people with normal intelligence for love and care in normal daily life. Many parents may reject or show reluctance in having children with limited intelligence. They may consciously or unconsciously pay more attention or cast more hope on other children with normal intelligence and good performance, in which they may thus neglect their child with an intellectual disability and deprived him/her of their intimacy need. For those parents with good acceptance and intense love and concern for their children with intellectual disabilities, their family caregiving load is insurmountable, in particular those children with moderate or severe disabilities. They may burn out or have compassionate fatigue in which they cannot satisfy the prolonged intense intimacy need and dependence of children with intellectual disabilities.

In many cases, having children with intellectual disabilities may stir up or intensify all sorts of family dynamics, marital discord or sibling rivalry in the family. Under such family conditions, the caregiving and development of children with intellectual disabilities is greatly hindered and disturbed. Very often, it may result in deprivation of intimacy as well as abusive intimacy.

People with intellectual disabilities usually do not have full access to education, employment and related medical and social services to support their normal development in different life stages. Very often, they may even be labelled, looked down upon and even bullied by others in the community, school, employment or in service settings. In some case, this involves severe abuse, neglect or oppression. All these maltreatments may further complicate their interpersonal relationships, self-image, meaning of life, emotionality and social functioning. They may displace all these negative emotions in forms of SADE towards those supportive others, including family members and professionals. As a consequence, they may be afraid of staying close or even have further intimate relationships with people with intellectual disabilities.

Because of their limited intelligence, they may always be performing a taking role in intimacy relationship, in particular those with multiple disabilities and severe intellectual disabilities. It may add to the burden of the family caregivers as they grow older and consciously and unconsciously expect clients to be independent and even to take up a giving up to serve them.

They may have problem in expressing their needs for intimacy. They may be aware of others' readiness in serving their needs for intimacy. Under that condition, their regressive needs for holding or togetherness may be regarded by others as disturbing behaviours, in particular for those busy and overloaded caregivers.

They may simply express their needs for intimacy in forms of demanding physical intimacy, unable to express their needs for social, psychological, intellectual and spiritual intimacy.

INTIMACY AND AFFECTIVE BOND: IMPLICATIONS IN WORKING WITH CLIENTS WITH INTELLECTUAL DISABILITIES

Transaction, Social Network and Affective Bond

Within human relationships, according to the depth of interaction, there are three forms:

They are **transaction**, **social network** and **affective bond**.

Transaction

In transaction, both sides are engaged in formal interactions in which a formal exchange is ongoing. It can be a business, political, or a benefit-oriented deal in which either side urges for a fair and beneficial treatment. It is a self-interest-oriented interaction, where emotional involvement is minimal and rational calculation is the most important concern.

Social Network

The second form is social network in which people engage with one another within a network of relationships. Within the social network, there can be one-on-one social interactions, many-to-one, one-to-many and many-to-many social interactions. The density of the social network is how many human relationships are formed. Frequency is the number of interactions among members in the network. Intensity is the depth of interaction within the network. Duration is the how long the social interaction lasts.

However, relationships among members can be supportive or not supportive. There can be many types of combinations of different frequency, intensity, density and social support. For example, for those with high density and frequency but thin social support network, relation among members is superficial and self-interest oriented.

Affective Bond: Intimate Relationship

Affect bond is the most intimate relationship among related parties. It usually occurs within a family context, such as parent and child, husband and wife. It also occurs in other social contexts in which individuals regard others as important significant others.

Intimacy generally refers to the *feeling* of being in a close personal association and belonging together. It is a familiar and very close affective connection with another as a result of a bond that is formed through knowledge and experience of the other. Genuine intimacy in human relationships requires dialogue, transparency, vulnerability and reciprocity (Healthy Place, 2008).

Implications in Working with Clients with Intellectual Disabilities

For clients with intellectual disabilities, their exposure to opportunities in life is restricted by their limited intelligence. Thus, it is hard for them to engage in normal transactions and deal with others in business and political arenas.

As they may have problems in gaining a full normal employment and social life, their social network and related social support may also be restricted. Instead, they heavily rely on caregivers in taking care of them. The more severe the intellectual disability is, the more restricted in building up the ability in transaction and social network and the more they depend on intimate others in taking of them.

Nevertheless, for caregivers, in particular related workers in service units, only some of them may be willing to establish intimate relationships with clients with intellectual disabilities. Many of them may just regard professional intervention as a transaction in exchange for salary and professional status.

Despite all that, clients with intellectual disabilities still regard them as intimate figures they are heavily dependent on. That sort of empathic discrepancy is very common in service. It creates serious burdens in good and adequate professional care for clients with service delivery.

Contents and Depth of Intimacy

Intimacy and affective bond is the most important human relationship in our life. Within an intimate relationship, there should be several important contents in creating the depth of the intimacy. The first one is emotionality. That means, related parties can have vigorous, frequent and deep emotional exchanges with one another. There should be a deep emotional connection in understanding and supporting with one another. Secondly, there should be sustainable meaning in interacting with one another. In other words, individuals feel meaningful, constructive and beneficial in being close to one another. The final one is dignity in which members with an intimate relationship mutually respect one another. These three contents, *meaning, dignity and emotionality*, interact with one another within an intimate relationship. Relationships with all three elements should be a balanced intimacy. The deprivation of any one or two element implies that the intimacy is unbalanced and unhealthy. The depth of the affective bond or intimate relationship depends on the intensity, frequency and duration of mutual emotional exchange, respect, dignity and meaning among related members.

Implications in Working with Clients with Intellectual Disabilities

Because of limited intelligence, clients with intellectual disabilities have problems and difficulties in emotional expression and exchanges with others, in particular with their intimate caregivers. In additional to that, for them, meaning and dignity within intimacy are being cared for, loved and accompanied by their beloved caregivers. Any separation, leaving, death or abandonment by caregivers may mean shattering of meaning and dignity within intimacy of which is highly disastrous and traumatic for clients with intellectual disabilities. However, because of their limited intelligence, it is hard for them to narrate their worry, anger and loss. Instead, their unresolved negative emotions and traumatic experiences can only manifest in forms of severe, patterned and internal triggered self-harm, aggression, disturbing behaviours and emotional fluctuation (SADE).

The Structure of Intimacy

The *structure* of intimacy implies the infrastructure of intimate relationships, while *content* implies the depth of intimacy. Structure means necessary components to build up intimacy. It includes proximity, fusion, availability and affordability, as well as commitment. Without any one of these components, intimacy cannot be built. *Proximity* means how close related parties stay with one another. It is a kind of physical closeness ranging from physical touch or embracing to dialogue and eye contact. It also implies psychological and social proximity in which an individual feels alike psychologically and socially. The second one is *fusion* of a daily life pattern, emotionality and thinking, as well as personality among members. It is a kind of like-father-like-son articulation. The deeper the intimacy, the deeper the fusion between the two parties. The third one is *mutual commitment* among one another. Individuals are loyal, faithful and trustworthy to one another. The deeper the intimacy, the more complete the commitment. It is a kind of mutual commitment between husband and wife, father and son, as well as sister and brother. Commitment is more than mutual benefit and exchange. Instead, deep commitment is a kind of sacrifice for one another. Everyone takes other benefit more than his/her own. Finally, it is *affordability and availability* in which everyone is physically, emotionally, psychologically and socially available to others in intimate relationships. In doing so, individuals do not feel stressed. Instead, in being available, individuals feel happy and enjoy being companions and experience togetherness with one another. These four structural factors build up the infrastructure of intimacy. Only within this infrastructure, emotionality, dignity and meaning of intimacy can be accumulated, manifested and exercised.

Implications in Working with Clients with Intellectual Disabilities

For clients with intellectual disabilities, the infrastructure of intimate relationships should be the same as people with normal intelligence. They and their family caregivers also need fusion, commitment and proximity, as well as availability and affordability in intimacy. However, as restricted by their limited intelligence, these four elements manifest differently. For them, they demand physical proximity with their caregivers more than psychological, social and emotional proximity. Also, their commitment, fusion and availability exist in a straight direct way. Family caregivers demand a high commitment, deep fusion and long availability and heavy affordability. The discrepancies of interpretation and manifestation of fusion, commitment, proximity and availability, if not appropriately tackled, may make the family caregivers feel exhausted and uncomfortable. They need to be sensitive and appreciative to the straight-forward manifestation by clients with intellectual disabilities. For example, despite their limited intelligence, a person with severe intellectual disability can feel his caregiver's sickness and say simple words, such as 'sick' and give him/her a cup of warm water as a symbol of care and concern. Related caregivers should appreciate this symbolic representation of deep commitment, availability, fusion and proximity by the person with the intellectual disability.

Constructive versus Destructive Intimacy

Constructive means that the intimate relationship is beneficial and developmental to related members. Destructive intimacy implies the intimate relationship is harmful to related members. Constructive intimacy and destructive intimacy can be listed as follows:

Destructive Intimacy vs. Constructive Intimacy
One-Sided vs. Two-Sided Intimacy
Mutually-Respected vs. Dominating and Submissive Intimacy
Developmental vs. Manipulative Intimacy
Protective vs. Abusive Intimacy
Caring vs. Exploiting Intimacy

Within a destructive intimacy, it is one sided, dominating or submissive, highly manipulative, abusive and/or exploiting. Within a constructive intimacy, it is two sided, mutually respected, developmental, protective and caring. A constructive intimacy enables individuals a sense of love and being loved, hope and being hopeful, trust and being trustworthy. It is highly therapeutic in which individuals can gain a deep meaning of life even in times of suffering. It facilitates individuals to build a healthy self-system as well as a sound mind and body. As an opposite, destructive intimacy creates permanent harm to the mind, body, self-system and meaning of life. It is also the source of mental, emotional, physical, social and psychological problems.

Implications in Working with Clients with Intellectual Disabilities

Having a child with an intellectual disability is a lifelong high demand duty and obligation for family caregivers. Many of them are caring, protective, developmental and mutually respected of clients with intellectual disabilities. They try their very best to care, to nurture and to develop their children with intellectual disabilities. However, prolonged and heavy caregiving easily exhaustes family caregivers, in particular for those aged ones. With deteriorating physical conditions, they feel fatigue and no longer able to sustain the demanding caregiving. They need to put their children in institutional care. At first, they still can visit their children frequently and provide concern, support and care. They also welcome regular home leave for their children. Gradually, as their health condition deteriorates further, they cannot afford to take care of their children. In this stage, home leave and visits are finally terminated. For clients with intellectual disabilities, the gradual leaving of their beloved family caregivers is painful and unbearable. Their sense of abandonment can be manifested in forms of SADE.

There are also family caregivers who abandon their children with intellectual disabilities in their early age. Some clients may even transfer from one agency to another agency for accommodation service in their childhood, making them feel highly insecure and unsettled psychologically and emotionally. Unless they can build up good constant and stable attachment with caregivers in accommodation services, their sense of insecurity and abandonment anger can provoke them to have frequent SADE.

There are also family caregivers who manifest harmful and destructive intimate relationships with children with intellectual disabilities. They may physically or psychologically abuse, exploit, oppress or manipulate their child with an intellectual disability. Some may purposely manipulate their children so as to manipulate or display their anger and frustration towards their spouse, parent-in-law or other family members. For example, A is a client with an intellectual disability. His father committed adultery and abandoned his mother and him when A was fifteen years old. A's mother was highly furious and about that. From that time onward, she purposely abused and exploited A and made him sick. Whenever A was sick, she would phone A's father and demanded his immediate attention.

Manifestation of Intimate Relationships

In addition to content and structure, intimacy also has different types of manifestations. It implies how intimacy is being expressed, communicated and received by one another. Manifestation of intimacy includes the following:

- Physical intimacy is sensual *proximity* or being physically connected or togetherness with one another.
- Emotional intimacy implies emotional exchanges, sharing as well as connection and holding among members within an intimate relationship.
- Cognitive or intellectual intimacy implies exchanging thoughts, sharing ideas and enjoying similarities and differences between opinions in an open and comfortable way.
- Experiential intimacy occurs when two people get together to actively involve themselves with each other, probably saying very little to each other, not sharing any thoughts or many feelings, but being involved in mutual activities with one another. (Kakabadse

& Kakabadse, 2004; University of Florida, 2014; Lowndes, 1996; Giddens, 1990, Healthy Place, 2008)

Apart from that, there are also psychological intimacy, moral intimacy, social intimacy and spiritual intimacy. Psychological intimacy implies psychological closeness, including emotional connection and cognitive connection, as well as mental connection with others. Social intimacy is related social norms, social structures and inherent bonding in determining formal and informal relationships with others. Spiritual intimacy is sharing of similar religious beliefs, values and closeness within a religious organisation among members in an intimacy relationship. Finally, moral intimacy is the sharing of similar moral beliefs and values.

Implications in Working with Clients with Intellectual Disabilities

For clients with intellectual disabilities, because of their limited intelligence, it is hard for them to establish high levels of intimacy such as moral and psychological intimacy. Also, they are more inclined to rely on physical intimacy to manifest their need of emotional and psychological intimacy. Because of their limited intelligence, they are less able to understand and receive the psychological, emotional, moral and spiritual need from their caregivers and others with normal intelligence. That means, related caregivers also need to manifest their high level of intimate needs in a simple way. They should use physical closeness, touch, connection and togetherness to manifest their own spiritual, moral, emotional and psychological intimacy with clients with intellectual disabilities.

Affective Bond

Psychosocially, intimacy is manifested in forms of affective bond in which the individual is psychologically, socially and emotionally attached to his/her significant others, particularly in a parent–child relationship. Within the psychodynamic perspective, affective bond in the parent–child relationship can be described in terms of holding, attachment, pairing and following. In holding, the caregiver (parent) actively embraces and cares for the dependent (child). The prominent figure is Winnicott (1964, 1965). In attachment, the attachment object (child) actively attaches to the attachment figure (parent). That means, attachment figures simply play a passive role in delivering constant, stable and accessible attachment for the development and maturity of the attachment object. The key figure is Bowlby (1977). In pairing, both parents and children are in equal basis. Sullivan (1956) suggested an interpersonal view in which every human being, including parent and child, embrace an integrated tendency to relate to others. That means, both parties, caregivers and dependents, embrace equal initiates and needs to relate to others.

1. Holding (the caregiver has the highest authority, power, influence and responsibility towards the dependents).
2. Attachment (the dependent has high initiates and need to attach to caregiver).
3. Pairing (both the dependent and caregivers embrace equal need and initiates to relate to others).
4. Following (the caregivers have the lowest authority, power, influence and responsibility towards the dependents).

Winnicott's Holding and Holding Environment

Winnicott asserted that in the maturational process, the holding environment is of crucial importance (Winnicott, 1964, 1965). Holding implies both physical and social protection.

'Holding:

1. Protest from physiological insult
2. Takes account of the infant's skin sensitivity-touch, temperature, auditory sensitivity, visual sensitivity, sensitivity to falling and of the infant's lack of knowledge of existence of anything other than the self
3. It includes the **whole routine of care** throughout the day and night

4. The **minute day-to-day changes** belonging to the infant's growth and development, both physical and psychological…

Holding includes especially the physical holding of the infant, which is a form of loving….The mental health of the individual, in the sense of freedom from psychosis or liability to psychosis, is laid down by this maternal care, which when it goes well is scarcely noticed and is a continuation of the physiological provision that characterizes the prenatal state. This environment provision is also a continuation for the tissue aliveness and the functional health, which provides silent but vitally important ego-support'. (Winnicott, 1965: 49–50)

That means, according to Winnicott (1965), the holding environment is provided by the infant's mother in which she embraces him/her closely everywhere, giving him/her a feeling of security, being totally protected and connected physically and mentally connected with others. *When the infant is being held long and tight enough, s/he may develop a sense of security and being connected with others when s/he grows up. In other words, s/he assures that even when his/her mother leaves him/her for a short while,* sooner or later s/he will come back, and his/her love and concern is still there. S/he feels secure and connected. However, when the infant is not being held and tight enough, s/he may not able to develop a sense of security and being connected with others. Instead, s/he feels insecure and being excluded or separated by others. S/he needs the presence of others to maintain the superficial feeling of being together with others or not being excluded by others. A comprehensive articulation of the holding environment should involve actors, types of reciprocity and degrees of holding.

Actors in Holding

A. The holder
B. The being held

Types of Holding

C. Physical holding

D. Emotional holding
E. Social holding
F. Financial holding

Reciprocity of Holding

G. One-way holding
H. Two-way holding
I. Collective holding

Degree of Holding

J. Total holding and embracement and kiss
K. Holding and embracement
L. Embracing shoulder
M. Hand holding
N. Hand shaking
O. Non-aggressive punching
P. Give me five
Q. Touch

(Give and take towards different types of persons and different ages)

The holding needs by significant others is, in fact, a lifelong process demanded by everyone in every life stage.

a. Infancy (*prolonged and constant holding* with breastfeeding as well as full embracement whenever the baby needs and cries for help): holding as a sense of total existence and full sense of security (intensive physical, emotional, psychological and social holding by significant others)
b. Childhood (*regular holding* as sign of love and reward for doing good, as well as a sign for comfort in facing difficulties, traumas and suffering): holding as a sense of connection, ego relatedness (self-identity and self-image) as well as a sign of protection and comfort (moderate physical, emotional, psychological and social holding by significant others)

c. Adolescence (*occasional holding* as a sign of courtship and sex, a need for intimacy in deep friendships, recognition, emotional connection and self-affirmation) (mild physical, emotional, psychological and social holding by significant others)
d. Adulthood and Early Aging (*selective physical, emotional, psychological and social holding* as a sign of love, courtship and sex, a sign of comfort in time of facing difficulties, sorrow, trauma and suffering, a sign for deep connection, support and understanding) (Developing ability to provide for minors, children and subordinates)
e. Late Aging (*caring physical, emotional, psychological and social holding* as a sign of caregiving, concern, support, comfort and help)

In clinical practice, with family and parent–child dynamics, there are also deprivation, compensation, facilitation and manipulation in holding.

Deprivation, Compensation, Facilitation and Manipulation in Holding

1. Deprivation of holding need in a previous life stage may lead to compensate in later life stages. For example, an urge for regular and intensive holding even in adulthood
2. Intensive holding needs in times of difficulties, traumas, suffering and torture
3. Sufficiency vs. inadequacy
4. Care vs. manipulation in holding
5. Genuine vs. artificial holding
6. Suffocating holding vs. facilitating holding
7. Egocentric holding vs. altruistic holding
8. Mutual holding vs. one-sided holding

Implications in Working with Clients with Intellectual Disabilities

The holding environment, especially physical holding, is crucial in working with clients with intellectual disabilities. As previously mentioned, most of them harbour a strong need of being cared for and feel concern from their caregivers. The more severe their intellectual disability, the more they are dependent on their caregivers. Also, intellectually, they are children, and they demand intense holding. In clinical practice, those clients who suffered from abandonment trauma, deprivation of love and attachment are inclined to rely on physical holding by caregivers to gratify their intense attachment hunger. In Winnicott's terms, physical holding is a kind of deep emotional connection between mother and child. It is also a kind of regressive comfort for clients with intellectual disabilities.

Physical Holding Intervention for Clients with Intellectual Disabilities

As physical holding is so important for clients with intellectual disabilities, a physical holding intervention should include the following elements:

1. Related workers should believe and affirm that physical holding and touch are crucial in human engagement, in particular for those vulnerable, fragile and emotionally deprived clients such as people with intellectual disabilities.
2. Appropriate physical holding provided by caregivers has a strong unconscious touch in comforting, providing emotional concern, fulfilling attachment hunger and showing a deep sign of empathy and connection for clients with intellectual disabilities.
3. Related workers should beware of their own limitation, sensitivities, related unhealthy bodily experiences in life in providing physical holding for clients with intellectual disabilities. All these create burdens for professionals in providing appropriate physical holding for these clients.
4. Different workers may have different life experiences and interpretations of physical connection with others. Thus, they should understand, accept and cooperate with one another in providing different degrees and ways of physical holding for clients with intellectual disabilities.
5. For those clients with severe SADE, despite appearing to be highly disturbed, aggressive, stubborn and emotionally unstable, they still

aspire for care and concern. Behind SADE are unstable emotions, attachment hunger, abandonment anger and abandonment fear. Appropriate physical holding, very often, can serve as a symbolic gesture in comforting unstable emotions, gratifying attachment hunger, ironing abandonment anger and securing abandonment fear.

6. Physical aggression can be interpreted as negative manifestation of the need of physical intimacy. It is also a release of suppressed abandonment anger. Appropriate holding can serve as a physical prompting to hold up aggressive impulses. It can also channel suppressed anger in appropriate ways.
7. There are different manifestations of physical holding in intervention, including physical embracing, hand holding, sitting together, having a meal together and physical touch, as well as doing physical exercise such as running, martial arts and hiking together.
8. Clients with a history of physical abuse may show reluctance in physical touch and holding, for it may trigger related traumatic memories. However, once such traumatic fear is appropriately released and resolved, their hidden attachment hunger may push them to urge for physical touch and holding.

Below are case episodes in demonstrating how appropriate physical touch resolves SADE in clients with intellectual disabilities. Related parties' consensus using their stories for academic purposes were sought. For the sake of confidentiality, their personal identities and information were appropriately disguised.

Case Episode 1: Attachment Hunger Fulfilled by Adhesive Physical Connection

B was a youngster with mild-grade intellectual disability and moderate autism spectrum disorder. Her father abandoned her and her mother when she was only five years old. Her mother was depressive and sad after the divorce. From that time onward, B was deeply emotionally and psychologically deprived. Later, B was admitted to a hostel for clients with intellectual disabilities. She was anxious, emotionally unstable and cried in the hostel.

Soon, B emotionally attached to the social worker, M, there. Whenever M was in the hostel, B approached M and embraced her waist like a small regressive child. At first, M felt a bit reluctant and embarrassed about B's attachment behaviours. She tried to push B away. However, the stronger she pushed B away, the more intense B's urge to embrace M. Some frontline workers interpreted this as attention seeking. Others interpreted it as disturbing behaviours that should be stopped, restrained or even punished.

Under the supervision of the writer, M began to be aware of the importance of physical holding for B. In facing B's embrace, M actively embraced B too. In addition to this, M patted B warmly. Interestingly, after two months of constant and active holding, B's attachment hunger was gradually gratified, she was emotionally stable and began to have good concentration in task performance and learning. Her embracing need shifted to holding hand with M.

Four months later, M's holding intervention was reduced to patting and hand holding with B for a short while only. B became independent and active in interacting and relating with others in the hostel.

Case Episode 2: Changing Aggression to Physical Connection

C was a client with a moderate grade of intellectual disability. He was strong, energetic and social. His father died when he was a small boy. C's elder brother took care of him. C admired and highly identified with him. C's elder brother was rigid and a strict disciplinarian. Whenever, C was naughty, he might punish C by requiring him to do vigorous exercise such as doing push-ups. Later, he married and had two young kids. He was too busy to take care of C and sent him to a hostel for clients with intellectual disabilities. C felt lonely and anxious in the hostel life. Occasionally, his brother visited C. He was very excited and manifested aggressive behaviours by pushing others to do push-up exercises. If others refused, he would hit them on the head.

Related workers thought that C's aggressive behaviours needed to be warned and stopped immediately. They threated C to stop all that immediately or else he would be deferred to meet his brother. Once C heard, he was highly stimulated. He yelled and pushed the worker and rushed to open the door and insisted to go home immediately. As he was strong and powerful, it hurt workers and C was sent to the hospital immediately. Despite the psychiatric medication given, the situation was getting worse.

Under the clinical supervision of the writer, related workers began to realize that C's aggression was a representation of his intense attachment hunger and excitement in the reunion with his elder brother. Him forcing others to do push-up exercises was only a recall of his memories of togetherness with his brother.

With the advice of the writer, whenever C pushed others, related workers should embrace him and do push-ups together with C, in particular before regular visits of C's brother. It seemed that all this physical connection enabled C to recollect his evocative memories with his brother. He became emotionally stable and happy in meeting his brother.

Bowlby's Attachment

Definition

Bowlby (1977) asserted that attachment is a primary need of humans to be loved, cared for and nurtured by a constant figure. He defined attachment as:

> 'Attachment is a way of conceptualizing the propensity of human being to make strong affective bonds to particular others and of explaining the many forms of emotional distress and personality disturbance, including anxiety, anger, depression and emotional detachment, to which unwilling separation and loss give rise'. (Bowlby, 1977:201)

With good and constant attachment, a person feels safe, secure and is emotionally stable. It is crucial for infants, children and adolescents to have secure and constant attachment so to ensure a normal and healthy physical and psychological development process. Good and secure attachment involves four crucial elements:

1. Proximity: Physical closeness between attachment objects and figures;
2. Constancy and Stability: Regularity of attachment; and
3. Availability: Readiness of attachment figures in attachment.

Insecure Attachment and Attachment Behaviour

A person with insecure attachment may have a mixture of feelings towards their attachment figure. These feelings include intensive love and dependency, fear of rejection, irritability and vigilance (Holmes, 1993:57). To ensure attachment, an insecure person tries to cling to his or her unstable attachment figure as hard as possible by means of 'attachment behavior'.

> 'Attachment behavior refers to any of the various form of behavior that the person engages in from time to time to obtain or maintain a desired proximity'. (Bowlby, 1977: 270)

Attachment Bond and Dilemma

> 'Attachment bond refers to an enduring attachment which the child confines to very few'. (Bowlby, 1982: 670).

Attachment bond is based on very secure and enduring attachment. But attachment behaviour is simply a reaction to insecure attachment. It represents a fear of losing attachment. A child who does not discriminate clearly between those to whom he has an attachment bond and those toward whom he simply manifests attachment behaviour is likely to be severely disturbed (Bacal, 1990: 216). For Bowlby, the human dilemma turns on the central importance of an attachment that cannot be entirely reliable, must perforce be shared and will be lost eventually. In the process of human development, maturity depends on the capacity to separate from the attachment figure and to form new attachments (Holmes, 1993:70).

Types of Insecure Attachment

There are several types of insecure attachments described by Bowlby (1977, 1982). They are anxious attachment, compulsive self-reliance, compulsive caregivers and detachment. Bacal (1990) has a good summary of these four types of insecure attachments.

Types 1: Anxious Attachment

> 'People suffering from anxious attachment are chronically fearful that they may lose their attachment figure, and their threshold for manifesting attachment behavior is low. They are often described as overly dependent or immature, and they are likely to develop neurotic symptoms, such as depression or phobia under stress. (Bacal, 1990: 214)

In other words, persons have fear of losing their attachment figure. Thus, they may become immature and depressed or stressed in their emotions (Bowlby, 1969).

Types 2: Compulsive Self-Reliance

> 'Those who are compulsively self-reliant have had similar experience as children to those who manifest anxious attachment. Although this behavior is the opposite of anxious attachment, these people also yearn for love and support; however, their reaction has been to protect themselves from rejection or from having to be someone else's caretaker by withdrawing from close relationships. They take care of themselves under all circumstances. Their resentment is also displaced to weaker people, they tend to react to stress with psychosomatic symptoms or depression. (Bacal, 1990:215)

To escape from the fear of losing their attachment figure, people with compulsive self-reliance tend to withdraw from close and intimate relationships (Bowlby, 1973). They may even display this sort of fear and frustration to other weaker persons. It may be manifested in the form of psychosomatic symptoms or depression.

Type 3: Compulsive Caregiving

> 'Compulsive caregiving is a form of attachment behavior in which relationship may be close, but the affectional bond is always one sided. Like the compulsively self-reliant, compulsive caregivers do not seek anything from anyone but, unlike them, constantly extend their attention and concern to others—whether or not they are looking for it. ….Bowlby equates the compulsive caregivers with False self personality configuration described by Winnicott'. (Bacal, 1990: 216)

Within compulsive caregiving attachment, the development of a person's self and personality is manipulated and controlled by his or her caregivers or significant other (Bowlby, 1977). As a result, the person may have difficulties in developing his or her true self and ability to be independent.

Type 4: Detachment

> 'The emotionally detached individual, who is incapable of developing a stable affectional bond with anyone, is usually identified as a psychopathic and or hysterical personality. His childhood experience is usually one of early, ongoing maternal deprivation as well as of parental rejection in later childhood'. (Bacal, 1990:216)

According to Bowlby (1982), prolonged detachment from attachment figure may result in an incapability of developing a stable affectional bond with others. As a result, the individual may be highly isolated and prompt to have psychotic disorder.

Type 5: Separation, Loss and Anger

Facing the separation and loss from the attachment figures, an individual may have to undergo a process of adjustment and adaptation. Holmes (1993) summarised these four stages which includes:

> 'Stage 1: Numbing
>
> (The very earliest response to a sudden bereavement may be an apparent calmness based on emotional shutdown in which all feeling are suppressed, or reality denied, until the bereaved person is in a safe enough situation to let go a little) (Holmes, 1993: 83)
>
> Stage 2: Yearning, Searching and Anger
>
> (The search of the lost object includes physical restlessness and searching everywhere, hoping that their lost loved one may reappear. The person also goes over in their mind every detail of the events leading up to the loss. Anger also appears towards the outcome by being angry towards anyone who is responsible for the loss of the attached figure. Anger also direct towards potential comforter so as to come to terms with the loss figure) (Holmes, 1993: 84)
>
> Stage 3 & 4: Disorganization and Despair and Reorganization
>
> (Loss throws the inner worlds and life of the suffer into turmoil. All the assumptions and expectations which depended on the presence of the loved one are now thrown into question. The quasi-depressive state which marks the third stage of grief can be understood in facing the loss. The sufferer tried to reorganize his or her new life by seeking for a new attachment figure)' (Holmes, 1993:89)

Implication in Working with Clients with Intellectual Disabilities

From Attention Seeking to Attachment Need

Under the prevailing influence of behavioural control of challenging behaviours, many professionals wrongly regard a client's attachment needs as attention-seeking behaviours. In terms of attention seeking, as the more attention given, the more intense the behaviours become. Thus, it should be ignored.

However, clients' intense attachment needs, once being ignored, can be increased to attachment hunger. Because of their limited intelligence, intellectually disabled clients can manifest this in forms of self-harm *(As no one cares about me, I am so bad and worthless)*, aggression *(You are so bad, you do not care about me)*, disturbing behaviour *(I am so lonely and desperate, please look at me, please come along with me)* and/or emotional fluctuation *(I am so lonely, I am so angry, I am so fearful that no one cares about me. I am so anxious. What should I do?)* All this attachment-hunger-related SADE is further misinterpreted by related workers as challenging behaviours that should be threatened, controlled, medicated or hospitalised. It becomes an endless vicious circle, starting from misinterpretation of attachment need as attention seeking and ending up by increasing and uncontrollable SADE. In terms of the attachment theory, this need should be properly fulfilled.

Only be doing so can clients with intellectual disabilities be emotionally and psychologically mature and stable. Also, once the attachment need is gratified, clients will become more autonomous and independent, and the attachment-hunger-related SADE will gradually disappear.

Intense and Confusing Anxious Attachment

For clients with intellectual disabilities, many of them harbour anxious attachments, as they are frequently transferred from one type of service to another. Also, their family caregivers may not be able to take care of them for their whole life. Thus, they may be transferred into rehabilitation service units, such as sheltered workshops, day care centres and/or hostels for their rest of lives.

Their insufficiency or even deprivation of attachment and love turns into anxious attachment with family caregivers or workers in service units. The more severe the intellectual disability, the more intense the attachment and dependency on others. Thus, the more anxious their attachment need becomes.

Pushy Compulsive Caregiving

Occasionally, some may manifest compulsive caregiving in which they attempt to take care of others so that they can get close to others and fulfill their attachment needs in a paradoxical way. It usually appears for those clients with mild-grade intellectual disabilities and high social functioning. In some situations, their compulsive caregiving may appear in an inappropriate way, such as forcing others to follow their own ways, pushing others to receive their offer or disciplining others to obey orders and regulations in service units. Many workers simply regard these as disturbing behaviours or as challenging their authority as workers in the service units.

Pseudo Autistic Self-Reliance

For clients with intellectual disabilities and severe degrees of autism, their intense attachment needs and hunger may intermingle with their autistic features. In searching for substituted attachment figures, they may be highly selective. Also, they may need a long period of time to establish a secure attachment with a new attachment figure. Thus, even though they have intense attachment hunger, they may still appear as self-reliant.

Sullivan's Integrated Tendencies and Pairing

Epochs in Stages of Development in Life

In terms of interpersonal psychiatry, Sullivan (1952, 1956) affirmed that there is a strong, integrated tendency for every individual to relate and to pair up with others.

The need of pairing with others gradually manifests from late childhood and early adolescence. Sullivan explained six developmental stages called "epochs" or heuristic stages in development.

	Stages (Epochs)	Characteristics
1	Infancy (Birth–18 months)	Gratification of needs (From birth to about age one, the child begins the process of developing, but Sullivan did not emphasize the younger years to near the importance as Freud.)
2	Childhood (18 mo–6 yrs)	Delayed gratification (The development of speech and improved communication is key in this stage of development.)
3	Juvenile era 6–9 yrs)	Formation of peer group (The main focus as a juvenile is the need for playmates and the beginning of healthy socialization)
4	Preadolescence (9–12 yrs)	Developing relationships within same gender (During this stage, the child's ability to form a close relationship with a peer is the major focus. This relationship will later assist the child in feeling worthy and likable. Without this ability, forming the intimate relationships in late adolescence and adulthood will be difficult.)
	Stages (Epochs)	Characteristics
5	Early Adolescence (12–14 yrs)	Identity (The onset of puberty changes this need for friendship to a need for sexual expression. Self-worth will often become synonymous with sexual attractiveness and acceptance by opposite-sex peers.)
6	Late Adolescence (14–21 yrs)	Forming lasting, intimate relationships (The need for friendship and need for sexual expression get combined during late adolescence. In this stage a long-term relationship becomes the primary focus. Conflicts between parental control and self-expression are commonplace, and the overuse of selective inattention in previous stages can result in a skewed perception of the self and the world.)

(summarised from Sullivan (1953) by Heffiner, C. (2012) *Chapter 5: Section 6: Harry Stack Sullivan*, https://allpsych.com/personalitysynopsis).

Integrating Tendencies

Sullivan (1956) affirmed that there is the individual driving force (integrating tendency) in relating oneself with others in interpersonal transaction. Sullivan interpreted integrating tendencies and dynamisms in a rather 'subjective' meaning, in which the individuals concerned feel and frequently use them in dealing with daily interpersonal situations.

> 'An even more striking approach to defining integrating tendencies, motives, or drives is in terms of what so-called "individual" people feel about these goals... And finally, and somewhat more obscurely, integrating tendencies can be defined in terms of the factors that they make relevant ....since integrating tendencies pertain to the very tissue of

> life – to what goes on between people – you can understand that we can define them in terms of what the people concerned take seriously'. (Sullivan, 1956: 8)

Integrated Tendencies and Emotionality

Affective bond can also exist in forms of integrating tendencies in which the individuals are inclined to relate with others so as to achieve a better interpersonal situation (Sullivan, 1956).

> 'Integrated tendencies may be defined, first, in terms of their goals, so that one might say that an integrated tendency is that sort of nature in two or more people which caused them to engage in reaching such and such an end state, which incidentally sets up the situation in which such process can occur'. (Sullivan, 1956:7)

That means, Sullivan (1956) considered integrated tendencies as an inherent urge for humans to live within an interpersonal situation. Sullivan interpreted integrating tendencies in a 'subjective' manner, in which the individuals concerned feel and frequently use them in dealing with daily interpersonal situations.

Integrated tendencies are a situation where two or more people engage with one another. It is both a goal as well as a process in which people attain to relate to one another. It is also an inherent tendency and inclination for human beings to interact, attain intimacy, understand and be understood, love and to be loved, as well as accept and to be accepted (Sullivan, 1959). *While emotional bonding refers to the emotional involvement with one's significant others, the holding and facilitating environment refers to the close and engaging social cycle that nurtures and supports the individual; integrated tendencies mean the individual's urges and inherent inclinations to related with others.* As human beings are social animals, each individual is related to many individuals in his various social cycles. While one may have a strong integrated tendency with his/her parents, s/he may only have a weak integrated tendency with his/her colleagues. The situation is even complicated while two individuals have different degrees of integrated tendencies in relating with one another. One has a strong tendency, but the other one has a low tendency. Instead, s/he may have a strong tendency to integrate with another individual. There may be four possible situations in manifesting one's (A) urge to relate with another individual (B).

1. Both A and B have strong integrated tendencies with one another.
2. A has a strong integrated tendency with B, but B has a low integrated tendency with A. Instead s/he has a strong tendency to integrate with C.
3. Both A and B have a low integrated tendency with one another. However, because of various reasons, they are required to live, work, educate and stay closely with one another.
4. Both A and B have a strong integrated tendency with C, but C has a low integrated tendency with them. A and B compete with one another for the integrated tendency of C to relate with him/her only.

All these situations have a strong impact on the emotionality of the individual. In the first situation, where A and B both have strong tendencies to relate to one another, the stronger the tendencies, the happier A and B will be, and the closer and more intimate the relationship between A and B is. For example, A and B fall in love and have strong tendencies to relate with one another. Under their strong integrated tendencies, they feel happy, satisfied and being in love in relating with one another. If their strong integrated tendencies can be prolonged and are not disturbed by external disturbance, their love and intimacy may be gradually intensified to a degree that they finally get married.

In the second situation, A has a strong integrated tendency with B, but B has a low integrated tendency with A. Instead s/he has a strong tendency to integrate with C. In that situation, there may be a highly confusing situation where A is unable to seek concern or relate to B. No matter how hard s/he tries or how much s/he tries to relate B, s/he is still ignored or neglected by B. Under that sort of condition, it is understandable that A will be deeply depressed, frustrated and lonely. B has a strong integrated tendency with C. If C has a strong integrated tendency with B, then both C and B will closely relate with one another happily and intimately. However, if C and B have different degrees of integrated tendencies, the situation will repeat again. That means, B may try all means to please C, but C would still have no intention or very low motivation to relate with B, making B highly frustrated, depressed and angry. Facing the relation between C and B, A's response is interesting. In C and B getting along well and relating with one another happily, A may become highly jealous and extremely angry with C to a degree s/he may take revenge, especially on C. However, if B cannot relate with C, A may feel happy, thinking that s/he still has chance to relate with B.

The third situation is a painful situation where both A and B have low integrated tendencies with one another. However, because of various reasons, they are required to live, work, educate and stay close with one another. In that situation, even though they are required to interact and communicate to accomplish tasks in daily living, working environment and other social contexts and occasion, they are mentally separated with one another. They may be apathetic with one another. They may also have conflicting views as well as unpleasant past experiences in encountering with one another. For example, within the same office in a company, colleagues may have to work and interact closely. However, related office politics and workplace bullying may make colleagues not only with low integrated tendencies have to relate with one another, but in extreme cases, they may even be angry or hate one another. Because of their low integrated tendencies or even negative feelings with one another, their togetherness may become a battlefield where they fight with one another in their work. The same thing happens in families where siblings, parents or couple are initially intimate partners with strong integrated tendencies to relate and interact with one another. However, family conflict, miscommunication, clash in personality, sibling rivalry, extramarital relationship, domestic violence and child abuse may make the family become a place for physical and psychological torture where family members with low integrated tendencies deal with one another but also try hard to avoid meeting one another, ending with traumatic experiences, torture, severe sadness, anger, jealousy, emptiness, frustration and loneliness.

In the fourth situation, both A and B have a strong integrated tendency with C, but C has a low integrated tendency with them. A and B compete with one another for C's integrated tendency to relate with him/her only. Within this situation, C may have different emotional responses. S/he may feel strange and bored in facing their competition for an intimate relationship. S/he may feel interested in manipulating the strong integrated tendencies of A or B to serve his/her egocentric desires. In the competition for a close relationship, A and B may be jealous and angry with each other. They may be highly sensitive to C's response towards them. Their emotions may be easily influenced by C's emotional response. If C shows acceptance to him/her, A or B may feel delighted and excited. If C shows rejection to him/her, A or B may feel depressed and unhappy. For example, both A and B fall in love with C, but C feels no interest to either one of them. A or B may try all means to arouse the C's attention, hoping that s/he can establish an intimate relationship with C. While they compete for the love of C, they may be jealous with one another and try all means to hinder one another in establishing an intimate relationship with C. Facing their competition for love and intimacy, C may feel highly bored, naive and meaningless.

A similar situation may occur in office setting, where both A and B compete for their close relationship with their senior, C, so that they can be appreciated and be promoted. They may try all means to arouse the attention of C, to show their loyalty to C, as well as to flatter C. In doing so, A and B may regard one another as competitors and be angry and jealous with one another. Facing the strong integrated tendencies of A and B, C may feel highly interested.

C may manipulate their dynamics to serve his/her egocentric desires and wishes. In doing so, s/he is selfish but feels happy, competent and contained in controlling and utilizing others. If both A and B cannot get their boss's appreciation after a prolonged trial, they may group together and transfer their anger towards C.

Integrated Tendencies, Dynamism and Self-System

In Sullivan's (1956) terms, integrated tendencies do not work alone; instead, it works together with the self-system and various dynamisms in various interpersonal situations. That means, the inherent urge of integrated tendencies is originated from the need of the self-system to relate and connect with others. However, in relating with others, there may be external hostility and anxiety. To protect the self-system and make the interpersonal situation still functional, various dynamisms are constructed by the individuals. Sullivan (1956) suggested that the self-system contains three important aspects:

1. The waking and active self (the active self);
2. The personality that is not readily accessible to self but self is the eccentric part (the eccentric self); and
3. The period in sleep in which the self is dormant (the sleeping self) (Sullivan, 1956: 4).

Sullivan (1956) suggested that dynamisms are formed so as to cope or misinterpret external hostility in maintaining the self-system within interpersonal situations.

> 'In avoiding or minimizing the anxiety that is inherent in the increasing struggle to protect the self system from the diffuse referential process that cannot be admitted into awareness, various specific processes, the dynamism, come into play'. (Sullivan, 1956: 4)

Gradually, the frequent recurrence of these dynamisms may result in problems in the self-system that lead to various mental disorders.

> 'Dynamism which we call dissociation is a mean of resolving the conflict between powerful needs and the restrictions which the self imposes upon the satisfaction of these needs'. (Sullivan, 1956: 6)

According to Sullivan (1956), integrated tendencies are an inherent urgency. This urgency can appear as a force, an internal force pulling individuals together. This force can be highly emotional in gratifying individuals' needs of intimacy, being loved and cared for. In pulling together, individuals can join together in attaining certain goals and activities. These activities may be ways to ensure the actualisation and maintenance of cohesiveness of the self-system. In doing so, these goal-directed activities and emotions driven together with others may be twisted and shifted in various forms of dynamism so that anxieties and hostilities in interpersonal interaction can be properly tackled, interpreted and articulated without challenging the integrity of the self-system.

Implications in Working with Clients with Intellectual Disabilities

An Unbalance of Integrated Tendencies

Because of limited intelligence, clients with intellectual disabilities tend to stay in the stage of childhood and preadolescence in which they are urging to be cared for and relate to others. They do not have enough capacity to relate with others as other adults with normal intelligence. However, the more they are unable to relate with others in a normal way, the stronger their integrated tendency becomes. Thus, in relating to others, especially with their caregivers, there may be an unbalance in integrated tendencies.

Different Situations of Integrated Tendencies

As previously mentioned, there may be four possible situations in manifesting one's (A) urge to relate with other individuals (B). If A is the client with an intellectual disability, B is the caregiver. These four situations occur differently in clients with intellectual disabilities.

1. Both A and B have strong integrated tendencies with one another. (This situation occurs when the family caregiver and the client mutually care for and love one another. The caregivers understand

the client's need deeply and facilitate the client to manifest the integrated tendency in an appropriate way.)

2. A has a strong integrated tendency with B, but B has a low integrated tendency with A. Instead s/he has a strong tendency to integrate with C. (This situation occurs when the family caregiver ignores or neglect his/her child with an intellectual disability. Instead, s/he cares and loves another child with normal intelligence. It makes the client feel inferior and neglected. Abandonment, anger and fear may manifest in forms of SADE. It also occurs in the service setting, and workers do not have good integrated tendencies to relate to intellectual disabled clients with intense attachment hunger, as they may manifested SADE. Instead, they like to relate to those social, emotionally and psychological stable clients who appear smart and lovely.)
3. Both A and B have a low integrated tendency with one another. However, because of various reasons, they are required to live, work, educate and stay close with one another. (This situation occurs when the professional caregivers or workers in service units do not care about the client with the intellectual disability. What they care about is only accountability, logistics, scheduled programs and structured activities in the service units. Gradually, clients with intellectual disabilities are unable to have good interactions and connections with workers. They simply live in the same service unit but with low integrated tendencies to know and relate with one another.)
4. Both A and B have a strong integrated tendency with C, but C has a low integrated tendency with them. A and B compete with one another for the integrated tendency of C to relate with him/her only. (This occurs when A and B are both children or clients with intellectual disabilities and C is the caregiver. That means both A and B compete for C's love and concern and manifest jealousy to one another. In this situation, SADE may occur between A and B.)

Integrated Tendency-Based Intervention

Within Sullivan's concept of integrated tendencies, interventions for clients with SADE should have the following features:

1. SADE may be a manifestation of unbalance integrated tendencies between caregivers, in which clients with intellectual disabilities have much stronger integrated tendencies than caregivers. The client tries to approach the caregiver, but s/he tends to ignore and neglect them;
2. As everyone embraces integrated tendency towards others in social life, it is important for caregivers to explore, identify and appreciate client's strengths and attachment needs. S/he should enable clients to express and manifest his/her integrated tendency towards others in an appropriate and acceptable way;
3. Clients' integrated tendencies are not limited to relating with caregivers; it should also extend to other aspects of life and interpersonal relationships. Thus, it is important for workers to facilitate clients to express their integrated tendencies with peers, neighbors and members in various social circles. Only by doing so, can clients lead normal lives within their own communities;
4. While emotional bonding refers to the emotional involvement with one's significant others, a holding and facilitating environment refers to the close and engaging social cycle that nurtures and supports the individual. Integrated tendencies mean the individual's urges and inherent inclination to related with others. In other words, within the concept of integrated tendencies, the client's and caregiver's relation and social interaction are performed in an equal basis. That means, while the client harbours a strong need to attach to the caregiver on one hand, on the other hand, the caregiver also enjoys and needs the companionship and togetherness with the client.

Kohut's Self-Object Relation and Following)

Kohut's self-object relationship has several components: the self, self-object, and the relationship between the self and the self-object.

Object, Self-Object, Self and Self-Object Relation

> In Kohut's terms, there are several types of objects, the need-satisfying objects, true objects and part object. Rycroft (1972) described that a need-satisfying object is an object that the subject 'loves' solely on account of its capacity to satisfy needs and whom the subject fails to recognise as a person. A true object is an object that the subject recognises as being a person with similar rights, feelings and needs (Rycroft, 1972:102). A part object is only a part of a person. (Rycroft, 1972)

Self-object

Kohut described a self-object as an object that we may experience as part of ourselves. There are two types of self-objects that respond to one's grandiose and idealised self.

> 'Those self-objects who respond to and confirm the child's innate sense of vigor, greatness and perfection; and those to whom the child can look up to and with whom he can merge as an image of calmness, infallibility and omnipotence'. (Kohut & Wolf, 1989:414)

These two types of self-objects are crucial in developing and maintaining the stability and equilibrium of the self. Strictly speaking, self-objects are neither self nor object; they are the subjective aspects of function performed by the relationship (Wolf, 1985:27). Consequently, the expected control over such an object is closer to the sense of control that an adult usually expects to have over his or her own body and mind rather than to the kind of control we usually expect to have over others (Kohut and Wolf, 1978). Bacal (1990) identified the following seven important functions for the *self-object*:

1. Attunement to affective states;
2. Validation of subjective experience;
3. Temporary identification within rightness of patient's perception;
4. Affect containment;
5. Tension regulations;
6. Soothing, sustaining, organising or restoring a weakened sense of self disrupted by self-object failure; and
7. Recognition of uniqueness and creative potentials. (Bacal, 1990:260)

Self

Self is defined as a unit, cohesive in space and enduring in time, which is a centre of initiative and recipient of impression (Kohut, 1979: 400). It is a psychological structure. It is an enduring configuration associated with the experience of selfhood. It consists of a cluster of potentialities evoked and maintained by self-object relationship (Wolf, 1984:61). It is established at the point in analysis when the self-object and its functions have been transferred into psychological situations (Kohut, 1977). That means, for Kohut, the self is conceptualised in terms of its relationships with its self-object (Bacal, 1990:229).

Self-Object Relationship

Bacal (1990) defined the 'self-object relationship' as one in which a relatively stable sense of the object's availability as a self-object prevails (Bacal, 1990:231). It is also a self-psychology concerning the state of self. It embraces on object–relation perspective in which the relationship between the self and the self-object is understood to be of central importance for the state of self (Bacal, 1990:231). In other words, it focuses on the psychologically meaningful self-experience of the effects of interaction between the self and its self-object (Basch, 1974).

Forms and Transformation of Narcissism

Kohut presented two forms of narcissism. One system attempts to create a perfect self, a developmental stage where everything good, pleasant and perfect is experienced as belonging to the inside and everything bad as belonging to the outside; it is called the 'narcissistic self'. Another system is the 'omnipotent other' in which the individual tries to identify others as self-object to pair, mirror and model with. This is a form of primary narcissism (Kohut, 1966, Siegel, 1966).

In the transformation of primary narcissism, according to Kohut (1996) there are five important elements: creativity, empathy, transience, wisdom and humor.

Creativity in transformation of narcissism means the parental imago is creatively shaped, modified and even maximised by the individual according to his/her own fulfilled needs as well as his/her cultural and social background and experiences.

Empathy means that the individual tries to make the parental imago as part and extension of himself/herself. That means, the individual not only develops close and intimate relationships with the parental imago, s/he also assertively affirms that him/her has similar natures, ingredients and characteristics as the parental imago.

Transience is the acceptance of one's mortality and impermanence as well as constraints and limitations in relation to one's omnipotence with others. In the transformation of the parental imago, transience implies that the individual clearly admits his/her own limitations, constraints and deficiencies. The more one admits his/her shortfalls, the more s/he regards the importance of the parental imago to his/her own existence. Also, in terms of narcissism, transience can be interpreted as unique and stylish personal features that are distinct from others.

Wisdom is the acceptance of variation and a stable attitude towards life and world. In transformation of the parental imago, the individual may gradually regard the existence and presence of the parental imago as constant and stable in life. S/he also slowly transforms his/her own identity as the parental imago. In doing so, s/he may not only create refined details about the parental imago according to his/her own needs. S/he may even feel that s/he has special wisdom in knowing about his/her life. S/he feels that with the togetherness of the parental imago or transforms into his/her identity.

Humor is a kind of attitude of being at ease or laughing at one's own difficulties, constraints and morality. It works to achieve transience in an enlightening way. It is an inner symbol that one not only accepts his/her own limitation and difficulties but also harbours an inner drive to look down all related difficulties to work through them and to integrate them in the process of personal development. In the process in shifting his/her parental imago into his/her own self-identity.

Implications in Working with Clients with Intellectual Disabilities

For clients with limited intelligence, the concept of the self-object relation is most applicable in understanding intimacy of those with mild-grade or borderline intelligence. For those with severe and profound disabilities, they may not be smart enough to choose their own self-object or build up their parental imago, grandiose self and omnipotent others. For them, they are more inclined to intense holding or attachment. Thus, intimacy for mild-grade and borderline intelligence is expressed in a different way. They tend to follow their substituted attachment figure rather than sticking and attaching to them physically and emotionally.

1. They may regard their substituted attachment figures (SAFs) (omnipotent others) whom they try to pair with (following SAF everywhere), mirror with (try to assume one day they will like SAF) and model with (copy every behaviours from SAF).
2. The omnipotent others (SAF) usually embrace some charisma or special talents that the client is highly attracted to. In addition to that, there are also many others who are also attracted by SAF. It may be a good competition among one another to earn the closeness towards the SAF.
3. The SAF does not show special interest or provide holding to the client. Instead, s/he simply allow the client to follow him/her. Occasionally, s/he may show some minimal care or attention towards the client and make him feel very excited.

All these may be demonstrated in the following case episode. Related parties' consensus to use their stories for academic purpose is sought. For the sake of confidentiality, their personal identity and information are properly disguised.

Case Episode, the Charismatic Coach

D was an intellectually disabled client in a sheltered workshop. Compared to other clients in this service unit, he was smart, energetic and a bit hyperactive. He came from a broken family in which his mother died when he was only five. His father was a merchant in the mainland China who needed to travel a lot. D was under the care of his grandfather who was old and sick. Most of the time, D wandered around his neighborhood and got along with some bad guys in the park. When his grandfather died, his father could not take care of them. He was then admitted in a private hostel for clients with intellectual disabilities. In the daytime, he stayed in the nearby shelter workshop. Among clients with intellectual disabilities, he was clever and brilliant. He was also naughty and occasionally disturbing and aggressive. Whenever he was bored, he came along and bullied some small and weak ones, in particular those who were profoundly and severely disabled intellectually. He also liked to push others to follow his order. Related workers labelled D as troublemaker in the shelter workshop. Sometimes, he even sexually harassed female workers by patting their bottoms. All this was unacceptable to colleagues in the shelter workshop. They pushed D to have psychiatric consultation, and an antipsychotic drug was given to D. For six months, despite D's regularly psychiatric medication, his condition did not show much improvement. Instead, his sexual harassment behaviours increased.

Under the clinical supervision of the writer, related workers were facilitated to learn all D's aggressive and sexual harassment can be interpreted as a symbolic representation of intimate needs and attachment. D did not like to physically adhere to others. He simply liked to follow those workers or outsiders with talent and charisma. Under the advice of the writer, D was related to a recreational instructor who came to the workshop to teach clients to dance and play football. The coach was a young guy, strongly built and handsome. He was attractive to clients in the shelter workshop. Many followed them closely. D tried to follow this coach and caught his attention. He followed him everywhere and learnt how to dance well. He also followed this coach in running a marathon. Three months later, D's aggressive and harassing behaviours disappeared. Instead, he was smart, social and helpful in the shelter workshop.

Intimacy and SADE: Interpretation and Intervention

For clients with intellectual disabilities, they harbour a strong need for intimacy. Because of various reasons, some of them can gratify their needs for intimacy adequately. Some cannot do so. According to that, there are four types in clinical manifestation and intervention:

Type 1: With Full Gratification of Intimacy Need

As their needs for intimacy are adequately fulfilled, they are emotionally and mentally stable, with empathy and care for others. Also, they feel secure, contented and self-confident. Despite their intellectual disability, they can care about others with a suitable degree of connection and genuine response. They are also able to develop their own potentials, abilities and talents.

Implications to Services and Intervention

Given that their significant others can provide continuous care and concern, as well as getting good support from professionals and related service, they are free from emotional, mental and/or behavioural problems.

Type 2: Insufficient Gratification of Intimacy Need with Mild Disturbing Behaviour and/or Emotional Fluctuation

As their needs for intimacy are inadequately or insufficient fulfilled, they are emotionally and mentally unstable. However, they can still search for substituted attachment figures, such as teachers, peers, mentors or professionals to ask for intimacy and attachment. Apparently, they may be attention seeking, with some progressive and active attachment behaviours. When their attachment need cannot be recognised, there may be some mild form of disturbing behaviours or emotional fluctuation. They may appear a bit egocentric, urging for others' care without sufficient recognition of others' readiness or unable to have reciprocal care and empathy to their substituted attachment figure. Anyway, if their intimacy needs are temporarily gratified, they are emotionally and mentally stable. With good companionship with others, they still can develop their potentials, talents, abilities and strengths in life.

Implications to Services and Intervention

Given that they can be supported by their significant others and substituted attachment figures, their emotional and/or mental condition can still be barely stable. Occasionally, they can still have mild and moderate anxiety, depressive mood or behavioural problems, in particular when facing separation, leaving, death of primacy caregivers, inappropriate or harmful institutionalisation, punishment and abuse. Once, they can work through all these with the support and care from others, they still can recover to a normal and stable mental and emotional condition.

Type 3: Deprivation of Intimacy with SADE (Self-harm, Aggression, Disturbing Behaviours, and/or Emotional Fluctuation)

In this type, clients with intellectual disabilities usually encounter emotional neglect, abandonment, separation or mild abuse by their primary caregiver in their early stages of development in life. Their intimacy needs are strongly deprived and undermined. They harbour an intense need for intimacy and care. They are hungry for love and care from others. Most of them manifest intense SADE (self-harm, aggression, disturbing behaviours and emotional fluctuation). Self-harm can be interpreted as a sign of turning abandonment anger inwards *(I am not lovable, as I am abandonment by others)*. Aggression can be described as a symbol for turning abandonment anger outward *(Others are so bad, as they leave me and abandon me)*. Disturbing behaviours may mean a highly egocentric way in asking for love, urging for care and attention without considering others' needs and readiness *(I need urgently for care and love. At least, this substituted attachment figure loves me and cares about me. I am not lovable and being abandoned by others)*. Emotional fluctuation can be anxiety, sadness, anger and loneliness in facing separation, loss and abandonment.

A Note on Self-Induced Trauma and Service-Induced Trauma: A Vicious Circle

Clients with intellectual disabilities with SADE engage in self-induced trauma. The SADE invites further trouble and self-induced traumatic experience. Certainly, self-harm leads to bodily wounds that can be harmful for a whole life. Aggression also lead to further isolation and deprivation of intimacy and isolation or rejection by others. Severe disturbing behaviours may invite rejection and exclusion.

In many ways, the manifestation of SADE can be highly disturbing, annoying and challenging for caregivers, including family members and professionals. If they cannot understand or connect with the intense intimacy needs or be empathic with clients' deprivation of intimacy, all these self-induced traumas may end up with further service-induced or caregiver-induced trauma.

Related family caregivers and professional caregivers may manage, control, restrict, isolate, institutionalise, medicalise, exclude and even abuse so as to inhibit or stop SADE immediately with a sound excuse of avoiding harming oneself and others.

Implications to Intervention and Services

However, our clinical experiences show that a careful understanding of SADE and a gradual fulfillment with clients' intimacy needs with the following procedures can effectively reduce clients' SADE and enable clients to regain normal life development:

1. Have a holistic understanding on the details, process, context and content of SADE;
2. Induce immediate action and care to minimize harm and hurt to oneself and others and avoid inappropriate medication, restraints, exclusion and control;
3. Identify underlying meaning, purpose, function, emotion and unfulfilled needs for being loved, cared for, hopeful, trustworthy and purposeful behind SADE;
4. Explore the clients' life development in which why, how, what and when they were deprived of intimacy from their primary caregivers in infancy, childhood, adolescence, youth, adulthood and aging. In what the deprivation of intimacy influences leads to clients' development and manifestation of SADE. How SADE further worsens into self-induced trauma and service-induced trauma;
5. Facilitate related parties including family caregivers and professional workers to understand clients' intimacy needs underlying SADE. Acknowledge their effort and difficulties in facing SADE. Have a thorough understanding about the dynamics between family caregivers and clients with intellectual disabilities in facing the vicious circle of deprivation of intimacy, SADE, self-induced traumas, caregivers and service-induced trauma;
6. Encourage related parties to show concern, show love, provide suitable holding, togetherness, certainty, care and guidance for clients. Provide appropriate support and resources for related parties. Resolve related difficulties and burdens accordingly;
7. All these should be done constantly, regularly as well as gradually so that clients' deprivation for intimacy can be smoothly compensated and fulfilled.

A Further Articulation of Related Mental and Emotional Problems Behind SADE and Deprivation of Intimacy

Coupled with severe deprivation of intimacy and SADE are also manifestations of moderate to severe mental illness, such inclination to borderline condition, unstable affect, panic and hysterical outburst, uncontrollable anger, somatic complaint and symptoms, severe anxiety and tension, attachment behaviour and disorder, depression or delusive thoughts and obsessive talks and behaviours. All these mental symptoms may be diagnosed as mental disorders. Many practitioners at this stage may be inclined or totally rely on the medical model with a constant intake of various types of psychiatric medications. In some cases, it may lessen the SADE or related mental symptom manifestation by simply turning SADE into inertness, withdrawal and passivity. In some cases, medication may not have any effects of SADE due to deprivation of intimacy. In that case, related professionals and caregivers should put medication and medical treatment in the following position appropriately according to the psychosocial conditions of the clients.

1. It may be necessary for those with severe mental problems, but it is not sufficient in recovery. Instead, medical treatment and medication should be paired up with humanistic understanding and psychosocial intervention.
2. Medication is merely one of the alternatives. When psychosocial intervention can work well, medication and medical treatment should be regarded as the last alternative.
3. Side effects of medication are harmful and should be fully recognised by related parties, including clients, their family caregivers and professionals.
4. Some medications may have direct effects on related mental problems. Some may only have accumulated effects and indirect effects on related mental and emotional problems. For those indirect effects, medication is in fact unnecessary. Related parties should try their best in understanding and delivering psychosocial intervention rather than relying merely on medication.

5. Harmful and inappropriate medication and medical treatment should be avoided and stopped as soon as possible by related parties.
6. Related professionals should facilitate clients with intellectual disabilities to have a proper attitude and rights in taking proper or avoiding inappropriate or even harmful psychiatric medication. A good guidance of this can be seen from P. Deegan's (1995) 'Principles of Recovery Model Including Medication' from https://www.power2u.org/downloads/MedicationMeetingPacket.pdf

Intimacy-Based Intervention for Intellectually Disabled People with SADE

As previously mentioned, SADE in clients with intellectual disabilities is deeply influenced by insufficiency and deprivation of intimacy as well as abusive intimacy and traumatic intimacy. Thus, intimacy-based intervention should be the effective intervention for intellectually disabled clients with SADE. As a summary of the previous discussion, intimacy-based intervention should include the following strategies.

Interpretation of Intimate Relationship and SADE

Firstly, there should a detailed interpretation of intimate relationships between clients with intellectual disabilities and their related caregivers, including those in the family as well as those substitute attachment figures in service units. Every intimate relationship should be interpreted in terms of content, structure, degree and manifestation of intimacy. Secondly, there should be an articulation of clients' SADE in relation to client's intimacy condition. Related workers should recognise how insufficiency and deprivation of intimacy as well as abusive and traumatic intimacy contribute to the occurrence of SADE, including SSADE and SOSADE.

Intervention Strategies

Upon the interpretation of clients' SADE and intimate relationships, related intervention strategies can be implemented. There are three main types. The first one is psychosocial interventions with family caregivers. The second one is developing intimate relationships with substituted attachment figures. The third one is developing a social network of intimate relationships for clients.

Family Intervention

Family intervention is important in dealing with intellectual disabled clients with SADE. Having a child with an intellectual disability is a lifelong burden. Many parents feel shameful and try to reject their children with intellectual disabilities. Only some parents try their best to take care of their children with intellectual disabilities. However, as time goes by, they feel fatigued, frustrated and exhausted, in particular when they get old and have poor health conditions. They reach a breakpoint that they need put their children with intellectual disabilities in institutional care for the rest of their lives. In facing marital discord or family dynamics, some parents manipulate or abuse their children with intellectual disabilities so as to control and manipulate other family members or air out their frustration and anger in life. Some parents are lonely and try to fully enmesh with their children with intellectual disabilities. This imposes a negative influence on clients with intellectual disabilities. The problems and difficulties in intimacy and the parent–child affective bond further nurtures SADE. Thus, family intervention is needed. Briefly, it includes the following intervention strategies:

A. Family mutual support group can be organised to facilitate parents' mutual support and sharing of hardship, frustration and difficulties in taking care of children with intellectual disabilities. They can also share the practice wisdom in understanding and effective intervention in facing children's SADE.

B. Family activities and recreation should be organised for family caregivers and their children with intellectual disabilities. Many of them, because of prolonged heavy caregiving duties, are deprived of recreation, exercise and community participation. Good and integrated recreational activities can increase their community participation, refresh their exhausted bodies and minds, increase good interaction and communication among family members and connect with other family caregivers.
C. Family education program should be implemented in providing related knowledge and intervention strategies for family caregivers so that they can develop proper experience, competence and correct knowledge in understanding and intervening SADE from their children with intellectual disabilities
D. Family counselling should be provided to those stressful, manipulative, abusive and exhausted family caregivers. Most of them embrace traumas in various stages of life. They need support in facing endless and exhaustive caregiving. They need advice on how to face SADE. They need counselling or healing on their lifelong trauma. They need advice to face marital conflict and discord. They need insight to work through dynamics and dilemmas in family relationships. All this should be facilitated in family counselling by related professionals.

Intimacy Network Building and Coordination

The intimacy needs and caregiving for clients with intellectual disabilities is highly demanding and can never be fulfilled by a single caregiver. Very often, related workers know that being a substituted attachment figure and gratifying clients' attachment hunger resolves their SADE effectively. However, it would be too demanding for them to be the only substituted attachment figure. Thus, it is important to build an attachment or intimacy network for every client with an intellectual disability. Also, it is healthy and normalised for clients to connect with a network of different people rather than unhealthy sticking attachment to only a few attachment figures. There are a few intervention strategies in establishing and coordinating an intimacy or attachment network. They are an interpretation of intimacy among people around, establishing intimacy figures and maintaining a balanced optimal attachment network.

Interpretation of Intimacy among People: Intimacy Ladder

It is important to have an accurate interpretation of degrees of intimacy for people around the client with an intellectual disability. It is an intimate ladder consisting of different figures with various levels of intimacy with the client. It can be list as follows:

Types of Figures (Degrees of Intimacy: Intimacy Ladder)

1. Substituted attachment figure (100)
2. Best friend (50)
3. Ordinary friend (20)
4. People around (10)
5. Stranger (0)
6. Hated person (–20)
7. Enemy (–50)

Substituted attachment figure (SAF) is an irreplaceable person whose clients simply regard him/her as a substitution of intimate family members, such as parents, children, spouse and/or sibling. There are several features indicating the intensity of bonding and importance of a SAF:

a. Whenever SAF presents, the client feels secure, happy, contented and relaxed.
b. Whenever SAF is absent, the client feels insecure, unhappy, anxious, sad and lonely.
c. The client feels jealous and bitter if the SAF shows kindness and concern to others.

d. SADE may occur when SAF is absent or being ignored or neglected by SAF.
e. SADE decreases when SAF shows concern or is together with the client.

A mark of '100' is given to the SAF showing that it is a full gratification of the client's attachment and intimacy need.

Best friend means that the client can also stick to but is less influential to the client. S/he usually has good interaction and communication with the client. S/he also understand the need and emotion of the client, but s/he may not be so attractive and less important than the SAF. A mark of '50' is given to show that the presence of a best friend is important but not determining as SAF.

Ordinary friend means that the client is regarded as coming and going within activities, chatting and interaction. The presence of an ordinary friend can make the friend less boring, more interesting in daily life. But s/he fully recognises that the presence of an ordinary friend is on a come and go basis. A mark of '10' is given to show its limited influence on the client.

Hated persons means those being hated or disliked by the client. There are many reasons why the client hates them. It may be because of countertransference by projecting his/her anger or frustration on parental figures on this person. It may be due to some argument, conflict and frustration towards this person. It may be because of some interpersonal bullying being done. For some clients with intellectual disabilities, they choose some weak ones to display their life frustration on them. A mark of '–20' is given to show the degree of hatred feelings.

Enemies are certainly the most hated people the client feels. It may be those who humiliate, abuse or oppress the client for a long time. Very often, the client feels fearful, deeply dissociated, not recognised or depersonalised towards these figures. The appearance of this figure may provoke and trigger traumatic memories.

The classification and degree of intimacy of each type of figure can help related workers to have *an accurate estimation on the intimacy need* of the client.

For example, in the absence of an SAF, the client may feel dreadfully lonely and uncomfortable. It properly may lead to the occurrence of intimacy-lead SADE. Thus, it is important to arrange two best friends (50 x 2 = 100) to accompany the client so as to compensate for the absence of the SAF. In some extreme situation where no best friend can be found, it may be necessary to arrange ten ordinary friends (10 x 10 = 100) to interact with the client. However, related workers should fully be aware that two best friends or ten ordinary friends is only a temporary compensatory measure. They can never replace the importance of an SAF to the client.

Network Building and Development

As SAF is so important for clients with intellectual disabilities, it is important to develop at least two SAFs so that when one is absent, the other one can be present. Also, it is crucial to make the client have a spontaneous and continuous interaction and sharing among best friends in various social contexts, such as in groups, in a residential setting or in a supported employment. Contextual best friends can make clients feel supported and cared for in every social environment. Also, best friends within a social context means that they can have deep sharing on similar issues and events in every social context. Ordinary friends in terms of coming and going can be present randomly in related activities and contexts. They simply make the client adapt to group life and social interaction with others. Within network building and development, there are *three important intervention strategies.*

The first one is development of substituted attachment figure. Usually, it is better to nurture those 'best friends' and upgrade them to become SAF. There are several measures in doing so. The first one is ***proper use of evocative memory***. Winnicott (1965) mentioned an evocative memory is a good and warm memory with a holding figure. It can be memories of activities, interaction, physical and/social environment in being together with the SAF. In establishing a new SAF, the best friend figure should perform similar activities and do similar interactions as the previous SAF. In doing so, clients' evocative memories are activated. It gradually transforms the 'best friend' to SAF. However, the transformation is only temporary.

The second one is use of transitional objects. In a psychodynamic term, there are two types of objects: internal object and transitional object. Internal object implies the parental figure is being internalised into the mind of the child. So even when the parent is away, the internal object of the good mother is still crystallised in the child's mind. Thus, the child is psychologically and emotionally stable. Gradually, this internal object is the crux of maturity development of the child. The transitional object occurs when the internal object is not being crystallised. Thus, when parental figure is absent, the child needs to attach to transitional objects for a sense of security. Transitional objects can be soft toys, activities and interactions that bring back evocative memories. The effect of evocative memories can be served as transitional objects. In other words, when evocative memories are used by the 'best friend' of figures, the transitional object of the SAF is formulated. However, it is a temporary representation of the missing previous SAF. To formulate the permanent SAF, the 'best friend/temporary SAF' figure needs to have his/her own evocative memories with the client. Only when this unique evocative memory can be formulated, the internal object can be consolidated. All these can be demonstrated by the following case episode. Related parties' consensus to use their stories for academic purpose was sought. For the sake of confidentiality, personal identities and information was properly disguised.

Case Episode: Transferal of Substituted Attachment Figure (SAF)

F was a client with an intellectual disability. After the death of his beloved father, he was deeply attached to the worker K of the residential unit. However, K was going to resign from the agency. Knowing that K was going to leave the agency, K became mentally and emotionally unstable with the occasional occurrence of self-harm and aggression. Under the clinical supervision of the writer, the service unit began to have a transferal of SAF from E's 'best friend' figure. Worker M was chosen as the potential SAF for E. M began to do similar activities as what K did with E. They went to the same Chinese restaurant and had the same food as K did. They played basketball as what K did. After two months' time, E began to recognise M as a temporary SAF. To anchor his permanent SAF status, M began to develop his own evocative memories with E. M taught K to play tennis and martial arts. He also gave some special delicious food to E. Gradually, E internalised M's SAF position.

The third one is an upgrading figure in the intimate ladder. That means, an ordinary friend is upgraded to become best friend. Best friend is upgraded to become SAF. Appropriate upgrading has several advantages. Firstly, the client has already developed a good relationship with the figure. Secondly, in the process of upgrading, the readiness of related parties can be assessed. Thirdly, suitable figures can be chosen among related persons.

The fourth one is development of an intimate ladder in different social contexts. The first social context should be the family and relative ladder. The second ladder is the social service context. That means, that it is better to have two attachment figures. One is a primary attachment figure (PAF) from family, such as parents, elder sibling, uncles or aunts. One is the SAF from related workers in the service unit. The lower in the intimate ladder, the greater in number it should be. In other words, within each intimate ladder, there should one SAF, two best friends and four ordinary friends.

Maintenance and Coordination of Intimacy Network

After the intimacy network is developed, it is important for the worker to maintain his/her normal function. It can be constant review of the degree of intimacy among different figures with the client. It can be moving in new figures from ordinary friend, to best friend and finally to SAF. It can be an upgrading various figures in the intimacy ladder. It can be resolution conflict, dynamics and dilemmas within the ladder, especially in facing hated persons and enemies. It can vigorous intervention with abusive, manipulative and exploitative family caregivers. That means, a responsible worker should not fixate his/her status as SAF for the client. Instead, even SAF status is established, s/he should facilitate the client to develop a good ladder and network of attachment. S/he should develop new SAFs in service, a PAF from the family context.

Intrapersonal Intervention in Enhancing Intimacy

Family intervention and attachment network development are interpersonal intervention in enhancing intimacy. Apart from that, intrapersonal intervention should also be enhanced. Related intrapersonal interventions has been mentioned in content, structure, constructive intimacy, dynamics and power of intimacy. It includes the following:

- Use of physical holding and attachment;
- Following of charismatic leader;
- Balanced and unbalanced integrated tendencies;
- Awareness of anxious attachment, self-reliance, compulsive caregiving;
- Searching for caregivers in service units who are willing to develop intimate relationships rather than task-oriented transaction with clients; and
- Knowledge and understanding of the impact of insufficient intimacy, deprivation of intimacy, abusive intimacy and traumatic intimacy in causing various types of SADE.

All these should be worked together with a family intervention as well as an intervention in developing and maintaining an attachment network and intimate ladder.

CONCLUSION

As a conclusion, this chapter is a comprehensive discussion on intimacy and SADE in clients with intellectual disabilities. The writer described various features and natures of intimacy in clients with intellectual disabilities. The impact of intimacy on the occurrence of SADE are also depicted. Finally, various intervention strategies in enhancing intimacy for clients with intellectual disabilities is discussed. In fact, most clients with SADE are influenced by intimacy. It is common that SADE occurs within the following situations:

- SADE occurs before or after a client's home leave or family visit;
- SADE occurs when scheduled family visit or home leave is declined, delayed or changed;
- SADE occurs in separation, loss and abandonment of caregivers; or
- SADE occurs when family caregivers are highly manipulative, abusive, oppressive and exploitative.

All these clearly show that SADE is closely related to intimacy of clients with intellectual disabilities.

Chapter 5

TRAUMA AND RESILIENCE OF CLIENTS WITH INTELLECTUAL DISABILITIES: IMPLICATIONS IN INTERPRETATION AND INTERVENTION OF SADE

INTRODUCTION: TRAUMA AND SADE

Emotionality, intimacy and trauma are three crucial dimensions in understanding SADE in clients with intellectual disabilities. Emotionality and communication implies that SADE occurs simply as a way of communication and emotional ventilation. Usually, interactional-based SADE occurs only in an incidental way. Once, communication and intervention are facilitated, related SADE drastically disappears or may not happen again. Emotional-based SADE is usually highly patterned. Clients use SADE as a form of ventilation of unexpressed anger, fear or loneliness. Once related negative emotions are channeled and vented, related SADE can be decreased and minimised. In these two forms of SADE, external and situational factors in triggering and provoking SADE can be clearly identified and controlled.

Intimacy-based SADE is much more complicated than those, due to emotionality and communication, especially for those with deprivation and abusive intimacy; manifestation is intense, patterned, highly persistent and severe. It usually occurs when clients face separation, loss and abandonment, particularly before and after home leave or family visit, facing the death of family members, decline and change of home visit and family visit. In clinical practice, many clients with SADE, despite taking a strong dosage of psychiatric medication, still prevail and intensify unless their intimacy needs are properly fulfilled.

The most severe form of SADE is trauma-led SADE. Because of various reasons, many clients with intellectual disabilities with physical or psychological abuse by caregivers in families and service units. Because of their limited intelligence and communication abilities, they are unable to express or communicate all these traumatic experiences and memories. Instead, all these are dissociated and repressed. However, they can be easily triggered by in coming stimulus. When all these traumatic experiences and memories are recalled and rebounced, as clients' limited intelligence and communication deficit, they can only express all these in forms of severe and obsessive SADE, in particular self-harm and aggression. In communication, emotion and intimacy-based SADE, external and situational factors can be clearly identified and recognised. In trauma-led SADE, SADE is internally triggered. In most cases, external factors are hard to be identified. In this chapter, the writer will give a comprehensive review of nature, process and effect of traumas. Its implications in interpretation and intervention for intellectually disabled clients with trauma-led SADE are thoroughly discussed.

Service-Led Traumatisation of Intellectually Disabled Clients with SADE

In chapter 2, we have mentioned the case R, who was inappropriately handled by related workers. The fixation of behavioural control on challenging behaviours creates service-led traumatisation to the clients. Let us review the case narration again and map out the process of traumatisation on R. Related parties' consensus on using their stories for academic purpose was sought. For the sake of confidentiality, personal identities and information were properly disguised.

The Innocent Institutionalised Mental Patient: R

R was an adult client with an intellectual disability. He was born in a middle-class family in which his father was a teacher and his mother was a clerk in a shipping company. R had an elder brother and a young sister. In R's mother's pregnancy, related tests showed that he might suffer from an intellectual disability. His father insisted R's mother undergo an abortion, but she refused. As a committed Christian, she wanted to keep R. Thus, the giving birth of R became a conflicting issue between his parents. After R was born, despite him being intellectually disabled, he appeared as a lovely baby.

Two years later, R's sister was born. His mother quit her job to take care of R. Later, R's father was promoted as the headmaster in a primary school. While R's mother tried her best to take care of R, his father felt shameful to have a son with a moderate grade of intellectual disability. Emotionally, he detached with R. He did not accept R as his son. At home, he avoided talking and playing with R. Even though R's mother tried her best to encourage a father–son relationship, he was inert, passive and withdrawn in interacting with R. Occasionally, if R committed anything wrong at home, his father might become furious and impose physical punishment on R. At that moment, R's mother would come up and defend him. Because of that, R's parents had intensive quarrels about the caregiving of R. It made R very frustrated.

Despite his intellectual disability, he fully acknowledged that he was rejected by his father. Facing all that, R harboured intensive anger towards his father as well as towards himself. However, because of his limited intelligence, indeed, it was really hard for him to express all these complicated feelings. Instead, whenever, his father was present, this unresolved anger was triggered. To release his anger, he would hit and bump his head hard and frequently. Whenever his mother saw this, her heart was broken. She came forward and embraced R not to do so. However, her husband insisted that R was silly, retarded and hopeless and should be institutionalised in an asylum. When R heard that, he was so sad. He cried bitterly and bumped his head even harder. His mother was so sad and helpless in facing R's self-harm. Also, her husband pushed her very hard to put R into a boarding school for clients with intellectual disabilities. Finally, R was put into a boarding school for children with intellectual disabilities.

He stayed there for eight years. During this period of time, R's self-harm behaviours intensified. He bumped his head in the boarding school whenever he felt puzzled, confused or angry. Instead of understanding R's feeling behind his self-harm behavior, R was labelled as emotionally unstable. The social worker in the boarding school referred R for psychiatric treatment. Instead of understanding R's deep-seated self-directed anger in facing the rejection of this father, the psychiatrist simply diagnosed R with psychosis and required him to take antipsychotic medication. From that time onward, R was required to take antipsychotic medication. However, it did not help much for him to lessen his self-harm behaviour. Spontaneous bullying and isolation from his teachers in the boarding school made R not only committed in self-harm behaviours but also aggressive behaviours towards others. Whenever others rejected or bullied him, he might suddenly rush to the bully and bite him/her. After that, he went to the bathroom and bumped his head on the bathroom wall.

All these self-harm and aggressive attacks threatened both teachers and social workers in the boarding school. The frequency and intensity of the self-harm and biting others increased gradually. Very often, R would harm himself severely by causing his head to bleed. He also bit others seriously when he felt angry and confused. Related caregivers could do nothing to deter all these self-harm and aggressive behaviours. Caregivers in the boarding school tied R's hands whenever he tried to perform self-harm or aggressive behaviours. Finally, with his mother's consent, R was admitted to a mental hospital. From that time onward, R was hospitalised. R was frustrated by that. To ventilate his anger of being abandoned and detained in the mental hospital, at first, R was irritated and committed even more intensive self-harm and aggressive behaviours. Because of that, he was restrained in his bed for two days to deter self-harm and aggressive behaviours. In addition to that, he was injected with a heavy dosage of antipsychotic medication. Soon, all this made R became dull, inert and passive.

From R's case, it was clear that R was totally misunderstood by related parties including his parents, his teachers and medical professionals. They tended to neglect R's intense urge to be attached and accepted by his father. They did not understand that R had a hard time dealing with his father's rejection. They seemed to assume that R was intellectual disabled; thus, he did not have feelings of sadness and frustration as 'normal' people. They interpreted R's self-harm and aggressive behaviours simply as challenging behaviours induced by an intellectual disability. Instead of understanding the symbolic meaning and emotional needs behind all these self-harm and aggressive behaviours, they simply regarded that they were merely mental problems of R that should only be solved by continual psychiatric medication. Interestingly, even if R's self-harm and aggressive behaviours became worse even after continual medication, they still insisted that continual medication as well as hospitalisation was only way to manage and control R's self-harm and aggression.

From Abnormalisation to Traumatisation: The Stage of Development

From the previously mentioned case illustration, it is clear that R was undergoing a process of traumatisation by related parties. The process of traumatisation consists of several stages.

1. Ignorance of clients' unfulfilled attachment needs and their difficulties in emotional expression, ventilation and communications with others;
2. Abnormalisation of clients' struggle and symbolic ventilation of negative emotions of being rejected, isolated and ignorant;

3. Pathologicalisation of clients' struggle and symbolic negative emotion ventilation with labels, assessment and/or diagnosis of emotional, behavioural and/or mental problems;
4. Imposing involuntary and even coercive behavioural control, punishment, medication and hospitalisation to clients so as to inhibit their struggle and symbolic ventilation of negative emotions;
5. Neglect of the destructive and traumatic effects of imposed involuntary and coercive control, punishment, medication and hospitalisation on clients; and
6. Formation of a vicious circle of intensive self-harm and aggressive behaviours because of continuously being abandoned, misunderstood, labelled, medicated, institutionalised and rejected by caregivers as abnormal, pathological and untreatable.

Stage 1: Ignorance of Clients' Unfulfilled Attachment Needs and Their Difficulties in Emotional Expression, Ventilation and Communications with Others

In Stage 1, clients with intellectual disabilities are similar to R in harbouring a strong attachment need. They may be rejected by one of both of their parents. In some cases, it may be due to the fact that their parents are very busy and are unable to give sufficient attachment and caring their child. Because of their intellectual disability, in particular those with a moderate or a severe grade of mental retardation, they have difficulties in express their emotional and attachment needs. Thus, they may manifest some sort of attention-seeking behaviours or employ some symbolic way to express their negative emotions. When their anger of abandonment turns inward, they may exhibit different forms of self-harm behaviours. When their anger of abandonment turns outward, they may manifest different forms of aggressive behaviours. In some cases, other odd and bizarre behaviours such as collection or hoarding or unnecessary things always occur. In addition, some may turn into deep withdrawal and inertness, as their abandonment anger and fear cannot be expressed or ventilated. Instead, they need to suppress all these negative feelings. In doing so, their normal social functioning and social interaction are also inhibited.

Stage 2: Abnormalisation of Clients' Struggles and Symbolic Ventilation of Negative Emotions of Being Rejected, Isolated and Ignorant

In Stage 2, caregivers may be highly disturbed by clients' self-harm, aggressive behaviours, odd and bizarre behaviours as well as deep withdrawal and inertness. Instead of understanding clients' negative emotions and attachment needs and problematic behaviours, they tend to label all these as abnormal and difficult to understand and communicate. Some of them may try their best to make meaning of it. Some of them may feel helpless, fatigued and angry with the continuous and overloading with their family members with intellectual disabilities as well as self-harm, aggression and other emotional/mental problems. Coupled with the intensification from related marital problems and other family problems, related family caregivers may finally come to a conclusion that they do not have enough knowledge, courage, patience, skills, power or love to take care their family members with intellectual disabilities.

Stage 3: Pathologicalisation of Clients' Struggles and Symbolic Negative Emotion Ventilations with Labels, Assessment and/or Diagnosis of Emotional, Behavioural and/or Mental Problems

In Stage 3, the helpless, fatigued, angry and hopeless caregivers may seek help and ways to lessen their burden and explain and control clients' self-harm, aggression, emotional or behavioural problems. One of the most convenient ways for them to ease their plight is to seek the advice and consultation from professionals, in particular medical professionals. Under the influence of medical and deficit orientation, all these may be labelled and diagnosed as emotional and mental problems. To moralise these pathological labels, intellectually disabled clients with self-harm and aggression are diagnosed and assessed by psychologists or psychiatrists. All these diagnoses and assessment tools, despite that they may have good validity and reliability, only measures the clients' deficits, disorders or problems.

They fail to acknowledge clients' strengths, abilities and talents behind symptoms, problems and difficulties. They also fail to recognise clients' unfulfilled needs and wishes in attachment, interaction and communication with their significant others.

As they are pathological based and deficit oriented, all these assessments and labelling tend to show that clients with intellectual disabilities have poor chances of recovery. Their self-harm, aggression and emotional problems cannot be understood or explained psychosocially. The only alternative should behavioural control, time out and medical treatment, as well as institutionalisation and hospitalisation.

Stage 4: Imposing Involuntary and Even Coercive Behavioural Control, Punishment, Medication and Hospitalisation to Clients So as to Inhibit Their Struggle and Symbolic Ventilation of Negative Emotions

Thus in Stage 4, involuntary and even coercive behavioural control, punishment, medication and hospitalisation are imposed to clients so as to inhibit their struggle and symbolic ventilation of negative emotions. In the process, the needs, emotions, talents and strengths of the clients with intellectual disabilities are totally neglected. Instead, they are regarded as objects in transferring from one place to another place, from one type of institution to another type of institution, from one service setting to another service.

In the whole process, only clients' deficits, problems and difficulties are noted. Coercive detention and medication are moralised, justified, legalised and bureaucraticised by professional assessment and related ordinance as well as the helpless decision by caregivers, including family caregivers. In some cases, even medications have no effects on clients' self-harm, aggression or related problems; related parties still persist on inappropriate medication. In some extreme cases, clients with intellectual disabilities are detained in mental hospitals for many years without any traits or clear diagnosis of mental problems.

Stage 5: Neglect the Destructive and Traumatic Effects of Imposed Involuntary and Coercive Control, Punishment, Medication and Hospitalisation on Clients

In Stage 5, clients with intellectual disabilities have long been kept within coercive control, punishment, medication and hospitalisation for many years. However, the highly destructive and traumatic effects of all these harmful treatments are neglected by related caregivers, including professionals and family caregivers. In fact, the harmful side effects of psychiatric medication are ignored. For example, a client with autism with self-harm behaviours has to take antipsychiatric medication. Similarly, as he is abandoned by his family members, leaving him alone in the residential hostel, he cries bitterly. Then, related parties force him to take antidepressive medication. In addition, as he is nervous in facing residential care, he also needs to take antianxiety drugs. As a result, even though he does not have any symptoms of mental illness, he has to take nearly all major types of antipsychiatric drugs. It seems that related inappropriate harmful interventions such as coercive medication, involuntary admission and prolonged detention in mental hospitals simply become excuses for related professionals or caregivers showing that they have done some substantial measures for clients with intellectual disabilities. For some caregivers, even though they know prolonged detention is harmful to their family members with intellectual disabilities, they still adhere to this. They painfully regard it as the only way to alleviate their overloading and exhaustive caregiving of their family members with intellectual disabilities. Some even painfully accept that as the only way to avoid being hurt by their family members with intellectual disabilities and sudden outburst of violent behaviours.

Stage 6: Formation of a Vicious Circle of Intensive Self-Harm and Aggressive Behaviours Because of Continuously Being Abandoned, Misunderstood, Labelled, Medicated, Institutionalised and Rejected by Caregivers as Abnormal, Pathological and Untreatable

Finally, in Stage 6, it becomes an endless vicious circle of intensive self-harm and aggressive behaviours because of continuously being abandoned, misunderstood, labelled, medicated, institutionalised and rejected by caregivers as abnormal, pathological and untreatable. Some caregivers believe that all these are the most effective ways in dealing with clients' self-harm, aggression, emotional and mental problems. Some caregivers are fully acknowledged about the adverse effects of all these labelling, inappropriate medication and prolonged institution of clients with intellectual disabilities, but they have no way out. They are too exhausted, too lonely and too weak to take care of their intellectually disabled family members with self-harm, aggression, emotional and/or mental problems. Inappropriate medication and prolonged institutionalisation are the final alternative for them. All these dilemmas and paradoxes can be shown in the following case illustration by a family caregiver, Y. Related parties' consensus in using their stories for academic purpose was sought. For the sake of confidentiality, their personal identities and information are properly disguised.

> Y: My son was intellectual disabled. When he was young, I tried my best to take care of him. In his childhood and adolescence, he was a good son. Despite his intellectual disability, he knew how to follow my advice in taking good care of himself, and occasionally he cared about me. However, after he was admitted to a shelter workshop in a social welfare agency, he was bullied by his colleagues as well as instructors in the shelter workshop. He was very disturbed by all this unreasonable bullying and oppression. He wanted to throw his anger by fighting back on all this oppression. However, the more he intended to do so, the more he was bullied and oppressed.
>
> Occasionally, he was even bitten by the instructor of this shelter workshop. He had no way to ventilate his oppressed anger. The only thing he could do was to pass this anger towards me. When he returned home, he was highly irritable and easily broke into anger and violence. Sometime, even I when blamed him slightly, when I spoke too loudly, or when the environment was too noisy, he easily broke into anger and I sadly became the victim of his unpredictable violence and aggression. Once, I was seriously wounded and hospitalised.

Apart from being physically wounded, mentally, I was so depressed about the current situation. I knew sooner or later, my son might hit me again. How could I survive with this kind of life? When my physical wound was healed, I needed to consult a psychiatrist. He frankly told me the only thing I could do was to send my beloved son to a mental hospital to receive medical and hospital treatment. I had nowhere to go. It seemed that it was the only choice I could take. I asked related social workers around whether there was vacancy in residential care to care my son. But most of them had a long waiting list. Some of them refused to admit him, as he had an aggression record of serious aggression towards me. They labelled him as risky and could not be acceptable to his colleagues in residential life.

Under these conditions, I sadly sent my son to a mental hospital even though I knew he did not have mental problems. In fact, before he was sent to the mental hospital, a related social worker in the shelter workshop had already accompanied him for psychiatric treatment. According to the instruction of the psychiatrist, he had to take antipsychotic medication. In fact, he had taken it for two years already. Apart from being sleepy and inert in daily life, there was not any sign of improvement in his self-harm and aggressive behaviours, in particular after being bullied by others. Deep down in my heart, I knew that psychiatric medication and hospitalisation did not actually cure his problems. Rather, it was the only way to send the 'troublemaker' away. It was the only way that I could ensure my safety of not being hurt by my son's sudden outburst of anger and violent behaviours….Indeed, sending my son to the mental hospital was a painful decision.

From Y's self-narration, it was clear that as her son only had an intellectual ability, and it was always hard for him to express his internalised anger and frustration in facing bullying by others in appropriate ways. In no way could he contain it. Instead, even a small clue and stimulus in the psychosocial context may trigger the outburst of all this deeply canned anger and frustration in forms of violence and aggressive behaviours towards his mother. In addition, in the process of being bullied and mistreated, he also learnt this as ways to display his frustration and anger. Under that condition, Y became the victim of her son's angry outburst of violence and aggressive behaviours. In other words, people in the shelter workshop bullied and hit Y's son. Then he bullied and hit his mother.

Conceptual Underpinning of Trauma: Destructive Effects and Impacts on People with Intellectual Disabilities

Traumatic Event Defined in DSM IV

There are many definitions of traumas. In DSM IV, traumatic events are defined as follows:

> 'Traumatic events that are experienced directly include, but are not limited to military combat, violent personal assault (sex assault, physical attack, robbery, mugging, being kidnapped, being taken hostage, terrorist attack, torture, incarceration as a prisoner of war or in a concentration camp, natural or manmade disasters, severe automobile accidents or being diagnosed with a life threatening illness.
>
> For children, sexually traumatic events may include developmentally inappropriate sexual experiences without threatened or actual violence or injury.
>
> Witnessed events include, but are not limited to observing the serious injury or unnatural death of another person due to violent assault, serious accident, or disaster or unexpectedly witnessing a dead body or body parts.
>
> Events experienced by others that are learned about include, but are not limited to, violent personal assault, serious accident, or serious injury experienced by a family member or a close friend, or learning about a

sudden, unexpected death of a family member or a close friend, or learning that one's child has a life-threatening disease.

The trauma is especially serious and long lasting if the trauma is induced by others (torture, rape).

Re-experiencing of the traumatic event may be in forms of dreams, intrusive recollection, or dissociative flashback in seconds or even in hours'. (American Psychiatric Association, 1994: 443)

From the DSM IV definition, the following natures are described:

A: People Involved in Traumatic Event

A1: The Victim of the Trauma
A2: The Witness of the Trauma
A3: Victims' Significant Others Learn about the Trauma

B: Related Traumas Events
B1: Accidents
B2: Natural Disaster
B2: Warfare
B3: Personal Violence
(Physical Attack, Sex Assaults, Being Kidnapped)
B4: News about Terminal Illness

C: Duration of Traumas
C1: Short
C2: Long Lasting

D: Effects of Trauma
D1: Immediate Effect during the Traumas
D2: Re-bounce and Recall of Trauma
D3: Chronic Effect of Trauma

Traumatic Events of People with Intellectual Disabilities

In comparing people with normal intelligence, people with intellectual disabilities may be more vulnerable to the following traumas:

1. Maltreatment by caregivers, in particular, family caregivers;
2. Death of family caregivers;
3. Separation and neglect by caregivers; or
4. Witness of domestic violence.

Regarding the impacts of traumas, the resilience and communication of people with intellectual disabilities is less effective than people with normal intelligence. They are more vulnerable to hardships and sufferings in life, in particular, in the loss, neglect and maltreatment of family caregivers (Verdugo and Bermejo, 1997). Comparing with people with normal intelligence, the impacts of traumas may be more prolonged and long-lasting. As their communication abilities are greatly hindered by their limited intelligence, people with limited intelligence may not able to express and share their negative emotions and the rebounce of traumatic experiences. Some may even express in forms of sudden anger outbursts, self-harm and attack of others.

Acute Stress Disorder and Numbing in Facing Trauma

The destructive effects of traumas have three types:

D1: Immediate effect during the traumas
D2: Rebounce and recall of trauma
D3: Chronic effect of trauma

The immediate destructive effects of trauma is described as 'acute stress disorder' in DSM IV. The rebounce and recall of trauma is named as 'post-traumatic stress disorder'.

Acute Stress Disorder: Diagnosis, Symptoms and Etiology

The symptoms of acute stress disorder are described in DSM IV as follows:

A. The person has been exposed to a traumatic event in which both of the following were present:
    a. a subjective sense of numbing, detachment, or absence of emotional responsiveness
    b. a reduction in awareness of his or her surroundings (e.g., being in a daze)
    c. derealization
    d. depersonalization
    e. dissociative amnesia (i.e., inability to recall an important aspects of the trauma)
B. Either while experiencing or after experiencing the distressing event, the individual has three (or more) of the following dissociative symptoms: recurrent image, thoughts, dreams, illusion
C. The traumatic event is persistently reexperienced in at least one of the following: recurrent images, thoughts, dreams, illusions, flashback episode, or a sense of relieving the experience, or distress on exposure to remember of the traumatic event.
D. Marked avoidance of stimuli that arouse recollections of the trauma (e.g., thoughts, feelings, conversations, activities, places, people).
E. Marked symptoms of anxiety or increased arousal (e.g., difficulty sleeping, irritability, poor concentration, hypervigilance, exaggerated startle response, motor resilience).
F. The disturbance causes clinically significant distress or impairment in social, occupational, or other important areas of functioning or impairs the individual's ability to pursuer some necessary task, such as obtaining necessary assistance or mobilizing personal resources by telling family members about the traumatic experience.
G. The disturbance lasts for a minimum of 3 days and a maximum of 4 weeks of the traumatic events
H. The disturbance is not due to the direct physiological effects of a substance (e.g., a drug of abuse, a medication) or a general medical

conditions, is not better accounted for by brief psychotic disorder, and is not merely an exacerbation of a pre-existing Axis I or Axis II disorder. (American Psychiatric Association, 1994: 324)

Associated features:

- Symptoms of despair and hopelessness may be experiences in acute stress disorder and may be sufficiently severe and persistent to meet criteria of major depressive disorder.
- Survivors of the trauma may have strong sense of guilt of another's death that leads to ignore of health and basic safety after the trauma. Impulsive and risk taking behavior may occur after the trauma.

Culture Features:

Many symptoms and response to trauma may be culturally bounded and defined.

Prevalence
It all depends on the severity and persistence of the trauma.

Course:
- Symptoms occur immediately during after the trauma, last for at least 2 days, and either resolve within 4 weeks after the conclusion of the traumatic event or the diagnosis is changed.
- When symptoms persist beyond 1 month, a diagnosis of post-traumatic stress disorder may be appropriate.
- The severity, duration, and proximity of an individual's exposure to the trauma tend to the most important factors in determining the likelihood of the development of this disorder.
(American Psychiatric Association, 1994: 324)

From the above-mentioned description, it is clear acute stress disorder is actually a numbing towards traumatic experiences in which the individual tries to survive within the trauma.

According to Yip (2013), the numbing is a kind of self-dissociation from traumatic experiences. According to the above-mentioned diagnosis, the numbing in traumatic experiences manifests in the following ways:

1. *Numbing of client's sense of mind* (difficulties in concentration, avoiding of recollection of memory in trauma). It is also a retardation of individual's cognitive processing of related message, image and information in the traumatic experiences.
2. *Numbing of client's sense of self* (dissociative amnesia, sometimes including self-identity, intensive sense of depersonalisation and loss of the sense of being a lively person).
3. *Numbing of client's sense of environment* (severe sense of derealization, reduction of awareness to environment including time, space, color and brightness). It is a retardation of related perception and reception of the fear from the traumatic and life-threatening environment.
4. *Numbing of client's sense of body* (retarded sense of pain and hurt and increase toleration of wound and hurt).
5. *Numbing of client's sense of growth* (fixation on traumatic experience and inability to grow and develop). It is also a retardation of one's ability to predict the future within traumatic experiences. (Yip, 2013)

The numbing of five senses in the self-dissociation mechanism means that the individual's detective, receptive and processing power within the traumatic experiences is greatly slowed down or even paralysed so that the destructive effects towards the self-system, mind and body are immediately reduced. In an extreme situation, the individual does not feel pain and fear. The fight or flight mechanism in avoiding fearful stimuli is replaced by a high-tolerance mechanism. It allows the individual to retain his/her minimal physical functioning so to survive within traumatically fearful experiences. Within dissociative traumatic fear, the fearful senses are numbed, temporarily retarded, but not permanently impaired. Intensive fear still penetrates into the mind, the self-system and the memories of the individual, but it is temporarily stored, suppressed and repressed. However, the numbing not only retards one's five senses in inhibiting the destructive effect or intensive fear and threat from environment, but it also temporarily retards the ego and social functioning of the individual. Immediately after the traumatic experience, the individual appears to be numbed and dissociated for a period of time without expression of intensive fear or traumatic suffering. That means, the individual still inhibits part of his/her ego and social functioning so as to save and ensure the integrity of the ego and self-system (Yip, 2013).

Implications to People with Intellectual Disabilities

For clients with intellectual disabilities, as mentioned above, the impacts of traumas may be more long-lasting, as their resilience and expression power are less effective than those with normal intelligence. That means, the numbing effects caused by related traumas may be more long-lasting. However, as people with intellectual disabilities are less expressive and interactive, the numbing effects may easily be ignored by related caregivers, in particular, those caregivers in institutions. They may wrongly regard clients' numbing as being peaceful and calm. Also, related traumas imposed by abusive caregivers, in particular, family caregivers are usually repeated one. They may experience repeated verbal or physical abuse, emotional neglect, prolonged abandonment and separation. All these repeated traumas tend to intensify the numbing effect imposed on people with intellectual disabilities. They gradually become inert, detached, dissociative and depersonalised in continuous and repeated traumas of abuse, neglect and maltreatment. Related traumatic memories and feelings are repressed and severely numbed. In some cases, related abusive caregivers may threaten people with intellectual disabilities to conceal related abuses. Coupled with their limited communication abilities, related traumatic memories and experiences are thus spontaneously repressed with a prolonged numbing.

Post-Traumatic Stress Disorder, Diagnosis, Symptoms and Etiology

As the individual ego and social functioning return to normal, the stored, suppressed or repressed traumatic dissociative fear rebounds. The reassociation of repressed and dissociative traumatic fear implies that the mind, self-system and the body of the individual prepares to resolve and integrate the traumatic dissociative fear. The more traumatic the experience, the more powerful the rebound of the traumatic fear. In psychopathological terms, it is the post-traumatic stress disorder symptoms (Yip, 2013). According to DSM IV, they are listed as follows:

A. Person has been exposed to a traumatic event in which both the following were presents:
   1. the person experienced, witnessed, or was controlled with an event or events that involved actual or threatened death or serious injury, or a threat to the physical integrity of self or others.
   2. the person's response involved intense fear, helplessness, or horror (Note: in children, this may be expressed instead by disorganized of agitated behavior)

B. The traumatic event is persistently re-experienced in one or more of the following ways:
   1. *recurrent and intrusive distressing recollection of the event,* including images, thoughts or perceptions. Note: in young children, repetitive play may occur in which themes or aspects of the trauma are expected.
   2. recurrent distressing dreams of the events. Note: in children, here may be frightening dreams without recognizable content.
   3. acting or feeling as if the traumatic event were recurring (includes a sense of reliving the experience, illusions, hallucinations, and dissociative flashback episodes, including those that occur on awakening or when intoxicated) Note: in young children, trauma-specific reenactment may occur.
   4. intense psychological distress at exposure to internal or external cues that symbolize or resemble an aspect of the traumatic events.
   5. physiological reactivity on exposure to internal or external cues that symbolize or resemble an aspect of the traumatic events.

C. Persistent avoidance of stimuli associated with the trauma and numbing of general responsiveness (nor present before the trauma) as indicated by three or more of the following:
   1. efforts to avoid thoughts, feelings or conversations associated with the trauma.
   2. efforts to avoid activities, places or people that arouse recollections of the trauma.
   3. inability to recall an important aspect of the trauma.
   4. markedly diminished interest or participation in significant activities.
   5. feeling of detachment or estrangement from others.
   6. restricted range of affect (e.g., unable to have loving feeling).
   7. sense of a foreshortened future (e.g., does not expect to have a career, marriage, children, or a normal life span).

D. Persistent symptoms of increased arousal (not present before the trauma), as indicated by two or more of the following:
   1. difficulty falling or staying asleep
   2. irritability or outburst of anger
   3. difficulty concentrating
   4. hypervigilance
   5. exaggerated startle response

E. Duration of the disturbance (symptoms in criteria A, B, C and D) is more than 1 month.

F. The disturbance causes clinically significant distress or impairment in social, occupational, or other important areas of functioning.

Specific if
Acute: if duration of symptoms is less than 3 months
Chronic: if duration of symptoms is 3 months or more

Specific if
With **Delayed Onset**: if onset of symptoms is at least 3 months after the stressor (American Psychiatric Association, 1994: 425-7)

From all these listed symptoms, Yip (2013) affirmed that dissociative traumatic fear together with related experiences can rebound/reassociate in various forms of:

a. *full conscious rebounce*/reassociation (FCR) in forms of intrusive distressing recollection of events, including images, thought and perception
b. *full unconscious rebounce*/reassociation (FUR) in forms of distressing dream
c. *partial conscious rebounce*/reassociation (PCR) in forms of flashback, illusion, hallucinations and related episodes
d. *partial unconscious rebounce*/reassociation (PUR) in forms of psychological and/or psychological distress being triggered by external and internal clues that symbolise or resemble an aspect of the traumatic events

Chronic Effects of Trauma ADTR

According to post-traumatic stress disorder symptoms, chronic effects of trauma can be listed in terms of avoidance, dissociation, triggering and rebounce (ADTR)

- Avoidance: avoiding related stimuli, venue, time, context, persons, issues or narration
- Dissociation: suppression, repression and amnesia of traumatic memories and recall
- Triggering/Startle: hypervigilance, difficulties in concentration, difficulties in sleep, irritability
- Rebounce: full and partial conscious rebounce, full and partial unconscious rebounce

In ADTR, there can be different intensity, frequency and duration. ADTR is in different patterns in various types of traumas (traumatic loss, abandonment traumas, physical abuse, psychological abuse, incidental traumas and complex traumas).

In ADTR, it can be directly related to the trauma or indirectly related to (symbolic, metaphoric and paradoxically) trauma. ADTR in one trauma can be related to ADTR of another trauma.

Implication in Working with Clients with Intellectual Disabilities

ADTR also occurs in clients with intellectual disabilities in experiencing traumas. They may avoid related stimuli, place, venue, persons and context. In comparison with clients with normal intelligence, their avoidance may be more impulsive and dramatic. For those who have problems in communication and use of language, avoidance may manifest in a form of abrupt emotional fluctuation, as well as disturbing behaviours. Dissociation exists in suppression, repression and amnesia. Compared to people with normal intelligence, clients with intellectual disabilities may have a longer period of dissociation. Also, their dissociative effects can exist together with somatic symptoms, such as somatoform disorder, psychosomatic symptoms and/or health problems. Triggering exists in forms of hypervigilance, irritability, difficulties in concentration and sleeping. For clients with intellectual disabilities, because of limited intelligence and impaired ability to communicate and express their emotions, triggering can be more unpredictable and uncontrollable. For some clients, triggering can accompany with intense and prolonged catatonic stupor. Rebounce may be full and partial conscious ones or full or partial unconscious ones. For clients with intellectual disabilities, rebounce can be highly impulsive, destructive and intense. It can be uncontrollable self-harm and aggression. In fact, ADTR in clients with intellectual disabilities can exist in forms of internally triggered SADE. The following may illustrate this in detail. Related parties' consensus in using their stories for academic purpose was sought. For the sake of confidentiality, personal identities and information were properly disguised.

Case Episode: ADTR in Forms of SADE of a Client with an Intellectual Disability

F was a client with an intellectual disability as well as autism spectrum disorder. He was a client in a shelter workshop. He had problems in communication and expression his emotion. His father was very kind with him. He attached to his father closely. However, his mother was aggressive and abusive. Whenever she felt angry and F was naughty, she would beat him severely. Three years ago, F's father died.

> F's limited intelligence and impairment in the use of language made him unable to express his sadness and grief towards his father. From that time onward, whenever he looked sad and disturbed, he would bite his hand seriously. Sometimes the wound was so serious that he needed to go to the hospital. In addition to that, he might suddenly break into anger and pull female workers or clients' hair. In addition to that, he might suddenly turn angry and push others. Interestingly, whenever his favourite male worker appeared, he would calm down.

In terms of ADTR, F possessed two important traumas. The first one was traumatic loss of his beloved father. The second one was being physically abused by his mother. These two traumas combined with one another making F feel very annoyed. The loss of a good father in protecting and loving him made the physical abuse by his mother become more severe and unable. In the shelter workshop, he normally *avoided* female workers, in particular, those who appeared like his mother in age and figure. The biting of his own hand implied that he was in a stage of *triggering* of related memories and negative emotions in the death of his father. The aggressive behaviours of pulling female workers' hair could be regarded as a *rebounce* of anger towards his abusive mother. When his favourite male figure (substituted attachment figure) was present, all related traumas were suppressed and *dissociated.*

Delay of ADTR

Because of limited intelligence, the ADTR process in clients with intellectual disabilities are much delayed in comparison with people with normal intelligence. The more severe the degree of disability, the greater the degree of delay. While a normal person is able to react or respond to traumatic experiences, people with intellectual disabilities need a much longer time to process it. The delay of the ADTR, coupled with the difficulties in language use, is always a misunderstanding and empathic connection of intellectually disabled clients with SADE. For example, a client with severe intellectual disability is being bullied or threatened by a worker in a service unit. S/he may not able to process the trauma within the same day. Thus, s/he may not able to have any emotional response to the traumatic bullying in the same day, where other normal people can do so. However, after several days, in some cases, even after two weeks, the emotional response of anger is processed (rebounce). So, at that day, even when nothing unhappy is happening to him/her, s/he may still appear angry, frustrated and irritated. Under this condition, s/he may display his/her anger towards an unrelated other. The sudden outburst of angry aggression without any identified reason may make his/her family caregivers or caregivers in the service unit think that the client is unreasonable, uncontrollable and unpredictable. Under this condition, physical punishment or verbal threat is imposed on the client so as to deter his/her outburst of aggression. Unfortunately, this unhappy experience lays down a cause of delay rebounce of aggressive anger two weeks later. The endless cycle will go on, and the client will be labelled as having spontaneous aggression without any reasons. Caregivers may assume that medication can be the only cure.

Intimate Trauma and SADE in Clients with Intellectual Disabilities: Interpretation and Intervention

Abusive Intimacy, Severe SADE and Mental Problems

Many clients with intellectual disabilities encounter abusive intimacy. Their intimate caregivers abuse them. Within intimate relationship between clients and their family caregivers, there are engulfment, verbal abuse, physical abuse, enmeshment, overdemanding and manipulation, as well as oppression. Prolonged abusive intimacy has highly destructive effects on clients with intellectual disabilities. On one hand, clients with intellectual disabilities need to depend on their family caregivers for the inherent needs of intimacy. On the other hand, the closer they get to their caregivers, the more they are hurt and exploited within prolonged abusive intimacy. Abusive intimacy results in *severe SADE and/or related mental problems*, such as psychosis, major depressive disorder and borderline personality disorder.

Implications to Intervention and Service

Apart from inducing the previously mentioned intervention in dealing with SADE, severe SADE (SSADE) from abusive intimacies are even more complicated than SADE. Thus, the following should also be fully considered in related intervention and service for clients with intellectual disabilities and SSADE.

1. *SSADE-involved traumatic memories of abuse and oppression. It consists of intimacy crisis.* On one hand, the client urges for care and concern from others. On the other hand, intimate relationships and contact may arouse abusive and traumatic experiences. Thus, in actual intervention, even though related caregivers try to hold, to care and to embrace the client with SSAD, all these traumatic memories can be triggered and rebounce, in which the client appears as reluctant, resistant, and even confused. Some even have highly aggressive output towards the caregivers. Related caregivers need to protect themselves from all these sudden rebounce of abusive memories and aggressive output but still with enduring patience to insist on intimate care, concern and holding. When all these rebounces are dissolved by love and intimacy, the client begins to fulfill his/her needs of intimacy. However, in SADE because of deprivation of intimacy, the occurrence of intimacy crisis is mild or absent.
2. *Because of limited intelligence, clients may encounter problems in expression and communication with others. Thus, they embrace difficulties in expressing their traumatic experiences.* It is very hard for professionals to track back their abuse intimacy trauma in life. In some cases, SSADE may be externally triggered by smell, images, noise, touch, light and trivial objects from the immediate physical and social environment. In extreme cases, SSADE may also be internally triggered. Related professionals have to be very

cautious and sensitive in detecting and exploring clients' responses in SSADE. They should try their best to figure out the underlying psychosocial cause of SSADE and identify the possibility of abusive intimacy in clients' life development, in particular in infancy, childhood, adolescence and adulthood.

3. *Abusive intimacy usually comes from family caregivers, in particular parents. They may be exploitative, manipulative, engulfing, abusive and oppressive to clients with SSADE. However, they may cover up all these by appearing as polite, concerning and caring to clients with SSADE in front of others.* Related professionals may easily be disguised by their appearance and neglect the actual abusive intimacy imposed on the clients. Many of these intimate abuses and manipulations may not be consciously or purposefully imposed by the family caregivers. Instead, it may be due to pathological coping from marital conflict, rejection of taking caring of clients from other family members, family dynamics, personality and traumatic developmental history of family caregivers, overloading family caregiving duties and related mental problems. Facing all that, related professionals should first take an empathic stand in understanding family caregivers' caregiving load, difficulties and frustration in life, internal conflicts and personality, as well as family and marital conflicts and dynamics. Then, once the family caregivers are emotionally connected, they may be able to ease out their abusive intimacy towards clients. Under proper support and emotional connection, related professionals are able to help family caregivers to understand how clients' SSADE are related to abusive intimacy. With the help from empathic and supportive professionals, most of them may be willing to take an active step to develop healthy intimacy with clients. They are also facilitated to resolve their own difficulties and frustration in family and in life.
4. *In some cases, SSADE may be intensified by service-induced trauma.* Very often, related professionals are incompetent to handle clients SADE from intimacy deprivation. They ignore the

fact that clients regard them as substituted figures to fulfill their hunger for intimacy. The intense urge for intimacy and triggering of abandonment trauma nurtures the SADE. Related professionals simply impose behavioural restriction, control, restraints, medication and isolation for clients with SADE. Some, in particular those untrained workers, may use physical punishment or even physical or verbal abuse in response to clients' SADE. All these contribute to clients' *secondary abusive intimacy* with a result of SSADE and related mental problems. Thus, in facing clients' SSADE, primary and secondary abusive intimacy should be carefully explored. They should advocate for clients with intellectual disabilities in a supportive, humanistic and genuine service context so that they can be from service-induced trauma.

5. *Within SSADE originated from abusive intimacy, there are intense but unresolved fear and anger.* Intense and dissociative fear either represses traumatic memories developing a dissociative disorder or is triggered rebounce because of related stimuli from the immediate environment. Abuse anger is internalised together with repressed traumatic memories, making clients suffer from severe depression or psychosomatic symptoms. Abuse anger can be externalised in forms of intense aggression and destruction. Because of limited intelligence, clients may be unable to express their anger towards those who had abused them or they cannot project it outward. *Many of them simply use displacement to release their anger. That means, they simply choose anyone who is close to them or is unable to fight back to release their repressed anger in prolonged abusive intimacy.* Under that condition, family caregivers and related professionals, as well as other clients with intellectual disabilities, may become the victims of violence and aggression originated from displacement of anger in abusive intimacy. It is important that they can have a holistic view and profound understanding on clients' SSADE so that they can track back the source of anger from abusive anger. They should help clients with SSADE to release their anger properly. This should

provide clients with a secure social environment and gradually dissolve their traumatic memories through concern, love and care.

SSADE and Related Mental Disorders

Clients with SSADE suffer from trauma of physical abuse, verbal abuse, oppression or death and severe separation from family caregivers. All these traumas certainly have a profound effect on related mental problems of clients with SSADE. Generally, clinical practice and related theories show that different destructive effects of traumas may develop different types of mental illness, such as:

- Prolonged dissociative effects may result in dissociative disorders;
- Prolonged rebounce effects may result in panic attack and hysteria;
- Prolonged startle effects may result in severe generalised disorders;
- Prolonged breaking effects may result in delusive disorder as well as psychosis; and
- Prolonged loss effects may result in major depressive disorder.

All these can accompany SSADE for clients who suffer from abusive intimacy.

Prolonged Trauma, Severe Mental Problems and Severe Obsessive SADE (SOSADE)

Severe obsessive SADE (SOSADE) is the most severe form of SADE. In SSADE, intellectual disabled clients are triggered by external stimuli to rebounce their traumatic memories in the form of self-harm, aggression, disturbing behaviours and/or emotional disturbance. However, in SOSADE, the rebounce can be without external triggers. It can be done in forms of an internal trigger. Also, the rebounce can be highly regular and patterned, even out of the control of the client himself/herself.

Internal triggers and rebounce can appear in forms of continuous self-harm bumping or hitting one's hand continuously for hours. It can be sudden aggression towards someone without known course and external stimuli. It can manifest in crying painfully every morning. It can also be the inability to sleep for days with a result of quickly losing body weight. A deep look at the internal triggers of SOSADE can be due to the following reasons:

1. Related trauma, suffering and abuse are too severe that the clients with intellectual disabilities can never forget or suppressed. It can be regular rebounce so as to reduce the inner pain to a bearable level.
2. Related trauma, suffering and abuse occurs continuously, and while the old memories are suppressed and repressed, the new ones come. The new regular painful traumatic experiences become an autonomous trigger to the old ones.
3. The size of emotional containers of clients is too restricted to contain severe negative emotions coupling with the traumatic experiences. Thus, when the container is full of negative emotions, it simply overflows without any relationship to external triggers.
4. The hurt and traumatic experiences as well as negative emotions are so deeply compressed in the unconscious level. However, the longer it is repressed, the more difficult for the individual to be aware and control the rebounce of traumatic memories. It can rebounce in a partial unconscious way through non-declarative memories bodily response, such as uncontrollable fear towards bodily touch and smell or visual image in the environment. Very often, all these external stimuli are well embedded within daily social and physical environment making the rebounce highly habitual and regular in everyday life out of the awareness of intellectual disabled clients and their caregivers.
5. Clients with intellectual disabilities with restricted and limited ability to express, ventilate and manifest their compressed negative memories and emotions need a long period of time of regular and patterned daily release of all these compressed negative memories and emotions in the form of SOSADE.
6. Because of their limited intellectual disability, their processing of traumatic experiences, including memories, emotions, compression,

trigger and rebounce, are all much slower than those of people with normal intelligence. Under this condition, SOSADE may be interpreted as a very slow, bit by bit, long-term slow processing of related traumatic experiences, memories and emotions.

Implications to Intervention

1. It is a deep challenge for related professionals in facing internally triggered SOSADE. As they are highly regularised and patterned, related workers may find it hard to find the causes and understand related factors leading to self-harm, aggression, disturbing behaviours and emotional fluctuation. They may easily come to a conclusion that SADE has unresolved problems that can only be resolved by institutional control, medication, restraint or hospitalisation.
2. As SOSADE are highly regular, continuous, patterned and internally triggered, even an empathic stand or genuine holding and caring of professionals may not resolve or stop the outburst of the SADE. In some cases, because the physical holding may even trigger deep-seated abusive trauma, it may make the SOSADE even more intensive than regular outbursts of SADE. However a continuous regular holding and caring can gradually decrease the intensity, duration and frequency of SOSADE.
3. In other words, to resolve SOSADE, caring and holding should be done gradually, slowly, continuously and regularly.
4. There may be a complicated mechanism in resolving SOSADE, which can be summarised as follows:
   a. Having patience and tolerance to clients' SOSADE. Within a safe, secure, caring and supportive environment, allow the outbursts of SOSADE to go through a long period of caring and psychosocial intervention. Avoid unnecessary social control, medication and hospitalisation.
   b. Induce appropriate holding and caring with a psychological preparation that it may further trigger deep-seated and repression traumatic memories with a result of intensifying

intensity, frequency and duration of SADE. However, only in doing so, can the client clearly and thoroughly clean out traumatic memories that fuel future outbursts of SOSADE.

c. Only by a certain period of regular holding, acceptance and caring can the frequency, duration and intensity be gradually reduced but not diminished. During this period of time, related workers should hold on to a strong belief and faith in trusting that only constant, genuine and regular love, hope and caring can dissolve traumatic memories that lead to SOSADE.
d. When all these deep-seated traumatic memories and negative emotions are released through regular holding and caring and dissolved by love, hope and trust, clients' SOSADE gradually diminishes. However, it may arouse again but in less intensity, frequency and duration if clients encounter unpleasant experiences that are similar to former traumatic memories in nature.
e. When SOSADE diminishes, clients' intense need for care, holding and attachment may still exist that may firmly adhere to certain attachment figures, in particular, the caregiver who help them to go through the SOSADE recovery process. All these attachment needs may manifest in forms of mild disturbing behaviour or emotional fluctuation.

Case Episode: The Crying and Aggressive Traumatic Recall

All these can be demonstrated by the following case episode. Related parties' consensus in using their stories for academic purpose were sought. For the sake of confidentiality, their personal identities and information were properly disguised.

E was a client with a severe intellectual disability. She had been staying at the hostel for ten years already. Recently, she cried bitterly every morning in her dormitory for two hours. No special issues were found in provoking her outburst of sadness. Under the influence of the writer, they assumed that E needed care and concern to gratify her unfulfilled attachment need. Several frontline workers were assigned to embrace the client during her crying. However, E was highly irritated by the physical holding. Immediately, she used her sharp fingernails and scratched the hand of the worker. Despite their injury, they insisted on providing physical holding to E. To prevent further injury, they put on thick raincoats. They asked the writer for clinical advice and explanation. The writer advised them to take a detailed look at E's life history. It was discovered that E was abandoned by her parents when she was only five years old. They put E in a private hostel, which was poorly managed, and related workers continuously abused her. Whenever E cried bitterly, they put her in a dark room. E tried to struggle against this abusive treatment, but they tied her up, pushed her into the dark room and locked it up leaving E yelled and terribly shocked there. It was understandable that the physical embrace triggered E's traumatic memories and experiences of being tied up and locked up in the dark room. It also helped her to release all these dissociated and compressed traumatic memories within a caring and comforting physical holding. After two weeks of constant holding, E's outbursts of aggressive defence and struggle began to decrease gradually. At first, during the physical holding, her body was tense, anxious and struggled. After the release of all these traumatic memories, her body became soft and enjoyed others' embraces. Two months later, E's constant crying in the morning no longer appeared. Instead, she began to embrace the workers actively.

TRAUMA IN FAMILY CAREGIVERS

In having a child with an intellectual disability, parents may encounter various traumas in life. It can be listed out as follows:

1. Trauma in knowing the fetus may be subnormal in the pregnancy;
2. Trauma in giving birth of a child with an intellectual disability;
3. Trauma in acknowledging a developmental delay of the child with an intellectual disability;
4. Trauma in accepting the label of intellectual disability on the child;

5. Trauma in having conflicts with spouse and other family members in child-rearing and caregiving of the child with an intellectual disability;
6. Traumas in family caregiving of the child with an intellectual disability.
7. Traumas in facing the public labelling of the child with an intellectual disability;
8. Traumas in facing inappropriate or even harmful service, treatment and institutionalisation of the child with an intellectual disability;
9. Traumas in facing the future of the child with an intellectual disability; or
10. Traumas in facing the self-harm, aggression, disturbing behaviours and emotional disturbance.

In facing all these traumas in living and caring for the child with an intellectual disability, many parents or substituted family caregivers feel extremely exhausted, hopeless and meaningless. It is too easy to give up their family caregiving duties and make their child with an intellectual disability be institutionalised. Even if they are supportive, enduring and caring, despite all these traumas and sufferings, they are still afraid that one day when they die, their child will have no one to take care him/her.

Implications in Working with Clients with Intellectual Disabilities

In working with clients with intellectual disabilities, in particular those with trauma and intimacy-led SADE, related workers should be fully alert that related family caregivers all suffer from the previously mentioned traumas in having children with intellectual disabilities. Clients' SADE are closely connected to their parents' pathological resilience in facing their traumas in life. Thus, it is crucial that related workers should also provide family intervention in terms family support group and network and family counselling, as well as parent–child bonding and relationship enhancement for family caregivers.

In doing so, related workers should have deep empathy with the family caregivers, knowing that they have suffered a lot in taking care of their children with intellectual disabilities. Appropriate recognition, good alliance and empathetic connection is crucial in the intervention process. It is highly inappropriate in ignoring family caregivers' own suffering and just imposing demanding caregiving duties or requiring them to change their abusive, manipulative intimacy immediately. Only by recognising their caregiving burden, suffering in life-long traumas and helping them to resolve accumulated negative emotions can related workers gradually channel family caregivers to take care of intellectually disabled children with SADE in appropriate ways.

Trauma-Based Intervention for Clients with Intellectual Disabilities

Trauma-led SADE in clients with intellectual disabilities are the most difficult symptoms to deal with. It is internally triggered. It is highly complicated and intermingled with different forms of avoidance, dissociation, triggering and rebounce. Related intervention can consist of four levels: environmental intervention, interpersonal intervention and intrapersonal intervention.

Empathetic Discrepancy

Empathetic discrepancy implies that related workers fail to have good empathy in relating to clients with trauma-led SADE. Reasons behind this are listed as follows:

Difficulties, Stress and Trauma

Difficulties means that individuals can be resolved within his/her abilities and resources. In facing difficulties, individuals look at solutions.

In facing difficulties, an individual may enhance his/her concentration and productivity. A resolved difficulty is a challenge in upgrading one's talents and capacity. Stress implies an unresolved difficulty in which the individual looks for extra resources, comprehensive cognitive appraisal and extensive problem-solving skills and methods. In facing stress, individuals usually embrace a sense of anxiety, worry and helplessness. Once the stress is coped with and resolved, individuals retain their original status. However, trauma is unresolved stress that has an unbearably high intensity, high frequency and/or long duration. The determination of difficulties, stress and trauma is subjected to individuals' perceptions, coping abilities and available help within the social environment.

Because of limited intelligence and limited exposure in life, clients may have limited coping abilities and resources in facing difficulties, stress and trauma. There is a large discrepancy between clients with intellectual disabilities and their normal counterparts in coping. For a normal person, it is a difficulty. For a client with an intellectual disability, it can become a stress or trauma in life. This sort of difference easily becomes an empathetic discrepancy between workers and clients. While a caregiver regards it as difficulty or stress, the client can regard this as trauma. For example, in the leaving of aged parents, for normal people with good independent lives this may be regarded as stress. For a client with an intellectual disability who is still emotionally and psychologically dependent on their aged parents, their leaving certainly becomes an unbearable trauma.

Delayed ADTR

Empathic discrepancy also appears in the delay of ADTR in trauma. As previously mentioned, clients with intellectual disabilities usually have a substantial delay in ADTR in processing trauma. That sort of delay creates empathic discrepancies in which caregivers in the family and in service units do not consider the occurrence of SADE as a result of ADTR of previous traumatic experiences.

In addition to that, what make a stressful issue become traumatic can be unbearable intensity, frequency and or duration. It can also be linked to or intensified by other unhappy events. It can also be prolonged deprivation, demand, stress, unfair treatment, abuse and oppression from an unhealthy, demanding, deprived, oppressive and/or abusive psychosocial environment. It is easy to have empathy if the client suffers from trauma in high intensity, such as accident, physical abuse and/or disasters. However, for those traumas that are high in frequency and long duration, such as prolonged bullying or frequent neglect and rejection, it is hard for others including professionals to have appropriate empathy for the client. It is particularly serious in intervention with intellectually disabled clients having prolonged and/or frequent neglect or rejection by significant others in the family, work and community.

It is important that related professionals can embrace an appropriate empathy in understanding, interpretation and intervention of intellectually disabled clients with trauma-led SADE.

Internal Trigger of Trauma-Led SADE after Dissolving of Numbing and Dissociation

In severe and prolonged physical abuse, many clients with intellectual disabilities may be highly dissociated. The traumatic experiences and memories are deeply repressed. They may appear as a bit inert and withdrawal. This condition may be wrongly regarded by related caregivers as calm and emotionally stable, in particular when their related abuse or abusers are still present. The numbing and repression may be slowly and gradually dissolved by love, care and concern when clients are transferred to a supportive and caring service context. In many cases, after a long time (sometimes it can be six months or one year) being caring for by a supportive caring figure, related abusive traumatic memories rebounce gradually in forms of severe SADE towards caregivers and family members. This internally triggered and highly delay rebounce may be wrongly considered by clients' family members as being recently and continuously abused or maltreated by the current supportive service context.

Levels of Intervention

Intervention with trauma-led SADE can be divided into four levels:

Environmental Intervention

It is the establishment of a supportive, caring, secure and comfortable physical and social environment so that s/he would not be frequently traumatised and triggered. For intellectually disabled clients with trauma-led SADE, it is important that they can be removed from an abusive and/or oppressive situation to a supportive and caring family and service contexts so that that the harmful effects of related traumas can be ceased and minimised immediately.

Interpersonal Intervention

Interpersonal support is important to help the individual to go through and recover from traumatic experiences and have the feeling of being connected, cared for and loved; being there is crucial in generating clients' positive emotion, ego strengths, self-confidence, love, hope and trust to go through traumas in life and develop proper resilience. For clients with intellectual disabilities, it is crucial that the psychosocial intervention for trauma-led SADE should be done by their substituted attachment figures within a caring and support service or family context. That means, intimacy-based intervention should be implemented in resolving trauma-led SADE.

Intrapersonal Intervention among Different Traumas

Intrapersonal intervention enables clients to deal with the destructive effects of trauma.

It can be in two main directions. One deals with individual traumatic experiences and memories. Another one deals with relationships and a combination of various traumatic experiences in life. *There are five types of effects: the accumulative effect, the chain effect, the buffer effect, the primary and recency effects in describing the combined effects of various traumas in life.*

Accumulated effect means various traumas, T1, T2, T3 and T4 combine together. The destructive power is not because of T4, but rather a combined effect of T1, T2, T3 and T4. There must be some main theme in combining all these traumas. It can be similar negative emotion, social and physical context, persons, issues and stimuli that link up all these traumatic experiences in life. In the accumulative effect, *the healing should start with searching the main theme that connects with various traumas and tries to interrupt it by inserting happy and other recall.*

Chain effect means the related pathological resilience of a trauma becomes the leading cause of the next trauma. For example, in abandonment trauma, the client harbours intense attachment hunger that makes him/her quickly attach to another inappropriate or even harmful substituted attachment figure. Sooner or later, s/he will be abandoned by this harmful figure. *Within this, there should a strong unfulfilled need that absorbs client energy and addiction into the traumatic coping mechanism. Once this need is fulfilled, the chain can be broken.*

In the **buffer effect**, the individual usually can cope with the traumatic experience well. As the coping mechanism and related resources decrease, the individual may reach his/her final breakpoint in which the ADTR suddenly prevails. For example, a client with an intellectual disability copes with the death of her beloved father as her mother is alive. When her mother dies, her elder sister is still available to take care of her. When her elder sister dies, her younger sister can look after her. When her younger sister is the last resort, once she is married and fails to take of care her anymore, the client can no longer cope. Instead, the destructive effect of traumatic loss suddenly intensifies and prevails. In the buffer effect, the client usually has strong resilience. Once the resilience pattern can be regained, the healing can take place.

In the **primary effect**, the individual's trauma, usually severe and in early life, can have a profound influence on later issues in life. The healing is completed only when related memories in primary trauma in early life are resolved.

In the **recency effect**, the trauma occurs in recent time, making the client feel that its effects and influence are crucial and influential. The healing should begin in resolving the traumatic memory of recent events.

Intervention of Individual Traumatic Experiences and Memories

After the combined effect of different traumas in life are resolved, related caregivers can move to intervention of a client's individual traumatic experiences and memories. It can be an adjustment of unbearable frequency, intensity and duration. High intensity negative emotion in the rebounce of trauma is replaced by positive frequency and duration. In doing so, metaphor and symbolisation can be used. Body and mind can be shifted. For example, an intellectual disabled client is frequently triggered by memories and frustration in the traumatic loss of his beloved father. The startle and triggering effects of this traumatic loss push him to have frequent disturbing behaviours in the hostel. Apart from establishing a substituted attachment figure for him to replace the loss of his father, he is facilitated to participate in a group of drum playing. The rhythm of the drum can help him to air out his sadness, anger and frustration in this traumatic loss. Interestingly, after the regular attendance in this drum-playing class, all these trauma-led disturbing behaviours decrease drastically.

CONCLUSION

As a conclusion, this chapter is a comprehensive review of trauma-led SADE in clients with intellectual disabilities. The nature, effect and process of trauma are thoroughly discussed. Its implications in working with clients with intellectual disabilities are described. SSADE and SOSAE caused by abusive intimacy and traumatic intimacy are separately mentioned. Finally, trauma-based intervention strategies for clients with intellectual disabilities are suggested.

REFERENCES

American Psychiatric Association (2012) *Diagnostic and Statistical Manual of Mental Disorder V Edition*, Washington, D.C.: American Psychiatric Association.

Bacal, H. A., & Newman, K. M. (1990) *Theories of Object Relation*, Columbia: Columbia University Press.

Bowlby, J., (1977) 'The making and breaking of affectional bonds: Etiology and psychopathology in the light of attachment theory' *British Journal of Psychiatry*, 130: 201-210.

Bowlby, J., (1982) 'Attachment and loss: Retrospect and prospect' *Journal of American Orthopsychiatry*, 52: 666-578.

Carr, G., Horner, R. H., Turnbull, A. P., Sailor, W., Anderson, J. L., Albin, R. V. & Korgel, L. (2002) 'Positive behavior support: Evolution of an applied science', *Journal of Positive Behavior Interventions*, 4(1): 4 – 20.

Chan, J., Arnold, S., Webber, L., Riches, V., Parmeter, T. & Stancliffe, R. (2012) 'It is the time to drop the term challenging behavior', *Learning Disability Practice*, 15(5): 36-38.

Douglas, H. (2013). *Online Etymology Dictionary*. London: Longman.

Emerson, E. (1995). 'Challenging behaviour'. *Challenging Behaviour: Analysis and Intervention in People with Severe Learning Disabilities*. Cambridge: Cambridge University Press.

Giddens, A. (1990) *The Consequences of Modernity*, Blackwell Publishers Ltd.

Goffman, E. (1957) Characteristics of total institution in *Symposium of Preventive and Social Psychiatry,* 15-17.

Healthy Place (2008). *How to Develop Intimate Relationships?* HealthyPlace. HealthyPlace.com – Trusted Mental Health Information and Support - HealthyPlace.

Holmes, J., (1993) *John Bowlby and Attachment Theory*, London: Routledge.

Iacono T., Johnson H. (2004) 'Patients with disabilities and complex communication needs. The GP consultation'. *Aust Fam Physician* 33(8): 585-9.

Janseen, C. G. C., Schuengel, C. & Stolk, J. (2002) 'Understanding challenging behaviour in people with severe and profound intellectual disability: a stress-attachment model', *Journal of Intellectual Disability Research*, 46(3): 445- 453.

Kakabadse, A., Kakabadse, N. (2004) *Intimacy: International Survey of the Sex Lives of People at Work*, Basingstoke: Palgrave.

Lowndes, L. (1996) *How to Make Anyone Fall in Love with You*, London: Element.

Nirje, B. (1969). 'The Normalization Principle and its Human Management Implications'. In R. B. Kugel & W. Wolfensberger (Eds.) *Changing Patterns in Residential Services for the Mentally Retarded* Chapter 7, pp. 179-195 Washington DC: President's Committee on Mental Retardation.

Osburn, J. (1998). 'An overview of social role valorization theory'. *The International Social Role Valorization*, 3 (1), 7-12.

Ross, E. & Oliver C. (2002) 'The relationship between levels of mood, interest and pleasure and challenging behaviors in adults with severe and profound intellectual disability', *Journal of Intellectual Disability Research*, 46: 191-197.

Royal College of Psychiatry, British Psychological Society and Royal College of Speech and Language Therapist (2007) *Challenging Behavior: A Unified Approach*, Royal College of Psychiatry, London.

Scope about Disability (2010) *Challenging Behavior*, www.scope.org.uk/support/parents/challenging-behaviour.

Shannon, C. E. (2017). 'A Mathematical theory of communication)'. *Mathematics Harvard Education* 5:23-34.

Sullivan, H. J. (1953) *The Interpersonal Theory of Psychiatry*, New York: W. W. Norton & Company.

Sullivan, H. J. (1956) *Clinical Studies in Psychiatry*, New York: W. W. Norton & Company.

University of Florida (2014) *Physical Intimacy* Counseling.ufl.edu. Retrieved 2014-06-12.

Tuffrey-Wijne, I. & McEnhill, L. (2008) 'Communication difficulties and intellectual disability in end-of-life care', *International Journal of Palliative Nursing*, 14(4): 189-194.

Winnicott, D. W., (1964) *The Child Family and the Outside World*, London: Penguin Books.

Winnicott, D. W., (1965) *The Maturational Processes and the Facilitating Environment*, London: The Hogarth Press.

Wolfensberger, W. (1972). *The principle of normalization in human services.* Toronto, Canada: National Institute on Mental Retardation.

Wolfensberger, W. (1985). 'Social role valorization: A new insight, a new term, for normalization'. *Australian Association for the Mentally Retarded Journal*, 9(1): 4–11.

Yip, K. S (2012) *Emotionality and Mental Illness: A Multi-dimensional Model.* New York: Nova Science Publishers.

Yip, K. S. (2013) *Emotionality and Mental Illness: Volume I and II.* New York: Nova Science Publishers.

AUTHOR CONTACT INFORMATION

Kam-shing Yip
Professor, Department of Applied Social Studies,
Hong Kong Polytechnic University,
Hung Hom, Kowloon, Hong Kong

Email: kam-shing.yip@connect.polyu.hk

INDEX

A

B

C

E

F

J

K

L

Q

R

S

T